The Conspiracy of Aging

Fit & Sexy
— *after* —
Fifty

Ray Stern

RTR PUBLISHING
DALLAS, TEXAS

RTR PUBLISHING
4553 Keller Springs Road, Dallas, Texas 75248

Copyright © 1996 by Ray Stern.
All rights reserved. No part of this book may be reproduced or transmitted in any form or by any means, electronic or mechanical, including photocopying, recording or by any information storage and retrieval system, without the written permission of the publisher, except where permitted by law.

The suggestions for food, exercise, weight-training and all other health and/or fitness-related subjects in this book are not intended as a substitute for consultation with your nutritionist, fitness instructor or physician. Before embarking on any type of fitness program, you are advised to consult your physician or other qualified health professional for specific guidance. This book is not intended to replace professional medical advice. The author and publisher expressly disclaim any responsibility for any liability, loss or risk, personal or otherwise, which is incurred as a consequence, directly or indirectly, of the use and application of any of the contents of this book.

Publisher's Cataloging-in-Publication Data:

Stern, Ray.
    Fit and sexy after 50 : the conspiracy of aging and how to reverse / Ray Stern.
    p. cm.
    Includes bibliographical references and index.
    ISBN 0-9647526-0-3

    1. Aged--Health and hygiene. 2. Physical fitness. I. Title

RA777.6.284 1996   613.7'0446
    QBI95-20666

Printed in the United States of America.

00 99 98 97 96   5 4 3 2 1

BOOKS ARE AVAILABLE AT QUANTITY DISCOUNTS.
PLEASE CONTACT PREMIUM MARKETING DIVISION, RTR PUBLISHING,
4553 KELLER SPRINGS ROAD, DALLAS, TEXAS 75248.

*To my mother
and the memory
of my father*

Acknowledgements

This book could not have been written without the key contributions of several individuals. I'd like to thank:

Clare Stern, my wife, for her wisdom and support through the years; Bob DelMonteque, my best friend and inspiration; Monica Rios, my training partner and friend, for showing what results my philosophy can produce; Joe Weider, my longtime friend and guru, for all his help; Joe Gold and Armand Tanny, my mentors as a teenager; Bob Kennedy and Johnny Fitness, for their support; Lori Stapledon at the Life Extension Foundation for her invaluable help and research; Bruce Heather, for his valuable contribution to the chapter on drinking water; Dr. George Toledo, for his peerless plastic surgery knowledge and expertise; Martha Savelo and Marsha Friedman at Event Management Services, P.R. people extraordinaire; and Leslie Higgins Advertising of Fort Worth, TX, for their wonderful cover design.

And a special thanks to Benjamin Dover, Bill Sloan, and Jim Donovan for their writing, editing, and publishing expertise. Thanks, guys.

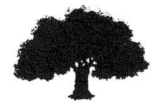

Contents

Acknowledgments

Foreword ... 1

CHAPTER 1
The Challenge and Conspiracy of Aging ... 3

CHAPTER 2
The Psychology of Staying Young ... 17

CHAPTER 3
My Own Story –
A Half-Century of Personal Research ... 31

CHAPTER 4
Diet and Nutrition for Health,
Long Life and Appearance ... 54

CHAPTER 5
Life-Saving and Life-Stretching Supplements ... 77

CHAPTER 6
Exercise and Fitness –
Why It's Easier Than You Think ... 87

CHAPTER 7
    Fiscal Fitness –
    What the Big Corporations Have Learned   **101**

CHAPTER 8
    Drugs to Slow Aging
    (and How to Get Around the FDA)   **112**

CHAPTER 9
    What Your Doctor Won't Tell You
    (Unless You Ask)   **130**

CHAPTER 10
    Plastic and Cosmetic Surgery – What to Expect **141**

CHAPTER 11
    Booze and Recreational Drugs–
    Are They Worth It?   **154**

CHAPTER 12
    The Shocking Truth About the Water You Drink **169**

CHAPTER 13
    Maintaining a Healthy, Active Sex Life
    to 100 or Beyond   **178**

CHAPTER 14
    Beware of the "Health Hucksters"   **189**

CHAPTER 15
    Rx for 100 (or More) Healthy, Happy Years   **198**

Bibliography   **213**

Index   **214**

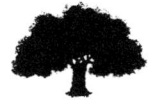

Foreword

I've known Ray Stern for a number of years -- both as a friend and as a doctor -- and I've always been deeply impressed with his dedication to physical fitness, his broad practical knowledge about the benefits of good nutrition, proper exercise and a healthy lifestyle, and his upbeat approach to life.

As a plastic surgeon whose goal is to help people look younger and more vital, feel better about themselves, and live fuller, more satisfying lives, it distresses me to see how many Americans allow themselves to grow "old" before their time. Modern medicine and science now make it possible for the years after age 50 to be the most rewarding, fulfilling, enjoyable time in our human existence. But far too many people fail to take advantage of the recent explosion in knowledge about the aging process and ways to counteract it. They fall into negative traps, some of their own making and others created by friends, family, government and society.

In this book, Ray Stern offers an "encyclopedia" of down-to-earth, common-sense information on feeling, looking and staying young. Using his own half-century program of personal self-improvement as a guide, he provides a wide array of "tools" -- ranging from the power of positive thinking to cosmetic surgery -- for keeping yourself fit, healthy, active, attractive and successful during your second 50 years.

Put into practice, the information in this book can not only stretch your lifespan; it can also change and enrich your years. It isn't the Fountain of Youth, but for millions of men and women in their 50s, 60s, 70s, 80s and beyond, it could prove to be the next best thing.

– *George A. Toledo, M.D.*

*"If we really want to live,
we'd better start at once to try;
If we don't it doesn't matter,
we'd better start to die."*
–W. H. Auden

CHAPTER

1

The Challenge and Conspiracy of Aging

A massive, monstrous conspiracy is afoot in our country today. Between now and the turn of the century, this conspiracy will kill more Americans than all the wars in our history put together. It will condemn millions more to a "living death" of needless disability and preventable disease. And it will make the so-called "golden years" of life a miserable, meaningless void for countless others.

If you're one of the tens of millions of U.S. citizens over age 50, you are the primary target of this conspiracy. If you're among the tens of millions of "baby boomers" rapidly approaching your 50th birthday, you're about to become the target.

The plot I'm talking about is silent, sinister and secretive. It's all around us. The chief co-conspirators in this plot are the very institutions we depend on for security, protection and assistance as we grow older – the federal government, the major pharmaceutical companies and major segments of the so-called health care industry.

A Scary Agenda

These powerful giants have their own special agenda for our over-50 population, and if you happen to be over 50, it's a pretty scary one.

The simple fact is, hospitals, clinics, nursing homes, medical labs and the vast network of companies that supply them with products and services have a vested interest in illness. So to begin with, let's stop calling them "health care providers" and call them what they really are – the "sickness industry." There's no profit for them in healthy, robust older people. They much prefer for us to be suffering from one or more chronic diseases – the kind that require numerous visits to the doctor's office, frequent hospital stays, endless tests and diagnostic procedures and lots and lots of prescription medicines.

The "sickness industry" doesn't like for us to argue or ask hard questions or express our own ideas and opinions. Its role is to make all the decisions about what's ailing us and what should be done about it. Our role is to shut up and take our medicine like good little old people.

But before I go any further, I want to make a couple of things very clear: First, when I refer to the "sickness industry" and the health care conspiracy, I'm not condemning all doctors or medical professionals – far from it. I don't want anyone to get the idea that I'm a "doctor-hater." I'm not. Certainly, there are many dedicated and enlightened physicians and surgeons who are genuinely concerned with their patients' wellbeing and quality of life.

A Dangerous Fallacy

I rely on the advice and professional expertise of a number of doctors, several of whom I consider close personal friends. And, in fact, several physicians have sought and followed my advice on matters of exercise, nutrition and overall fitness. I believe the right kind of medical care can not only promote healing and lengthen life but greatly enhance our after-50 years. As important as self-help and self-treatment is, there are times when it isn't enough, and at those times a doctor's services are essential. I would never advise anyone with a broken leg, for example, to try to set it himself, or someone with a raging infection to try to cure it on his own.

The trick is to know when to turn a problem over to the

doctor and when to take responsibility for it ourselves. The trick is to realize that having a regular physical exam doesn't automatically mean you're healthy – even if you pass it with flying colors. The doctor-patient relationship should always be a partnership, with the patient as an active participant, not merely a passive object to be poked, prodded, prescribed and given orders without explanation.

Too many of us persist in the idea that, whatever is wrong, the doctor will "fix it." This is a dangerous fallacy. We have to take responsibility for our own health. We have to demand the answers and information we deserve from our doctors. And we have to fight the tendency of some physicians to deal with human beings as if they were nothing more than widgets on an assembly line.

Everybody's a Specialist

The more complex medical science becomes, the more doctors become specialists. If you have foot problems, you see a podiatrist. If you have heart problems, you see a cardiologist. If you have an allergy, you see an allergenist. If you aren't sure what you have, you see a diagnostician. And so forth. This has produced a paradoxical situation. Today's doctors know more than ever about their own special areas, yet may know less about and be less concerned with the human machine as a whole.

In some ways, specialization is good for patients. It's good to know that the doctor treating your right arm knows everything there is to know about right arms. But don't assume the same doctor knows everything about your overall health or how to live a long, full life. His attention is focused on his own little piece of the good-health jigsaw puzzle. It's not his role to fit all the pieces together to form the big picture. The responsibility for "specializing" in the care of your entire body rests with you.

Very few physicians, for example, specialize in nutrition. Consequently, a doctor's office isn't the ideal place to go for sound nutritional advice. Only a small number of specialists in sports medicine are highly knowledgeable about the benefits of specific types of exercise. And except for a mere handful of medical trailblazers, don't expect doctors to recommend experimental or "unproven" drugs – no matter how great their potential benefits may be.

One of the biggest obstacles to making use of the effective new weapons against aging is the constant threat of malpractice lawsuits against physicians. If a doctor prescribes a drug that isn't approved by the FDA or a treatment that isn't sanctioned by the AMA, he vastly increases his risk of being sued. Insurance companies and the monolithic federal Medicare and Medicaid bureaucracies are another obstacle. They insist that certain blanket procedures be followed for certain illnesses, regardless of whether a specific patient needs such treatment or not. It all adds up to a costly, cumbersome, inefficient, depersonalized system.

Patients vs. "The System"

As wonderful as some individual doctors are, this system often makes their whole profession seem an insensitive, uncaring and money-driven machine. As modern medicine moves deeper into such complex areas as genetics and molecular biology, this problem is almost certain to grow worse. Scientists who see patients as mere collections of cells, chromosomes and molecules have a hard time seeing them as people. This is an unnerving trend. It promotes an environment in which patients serve science, rather than vice-versa.

And unfortunately, while some areas of science advance, other areas regress. Despite the huge advancements in our overall knowledge about food elements, vitamins, minerals and how they all work together in our bodies, many doctors and so-called "nutritionists" are still operating in the "dark ages" where diet is concerned. Why else would more than seven out of every ten Americans be overweight today – despite our huge strides in producing low-fat, low-calorie foods?

Our sophisticated, high-tech system of health care has a disturbing tendency to treat the symptoms of a specific illness and ignore the need to build and protect overall health. It's always easier to prescribe another pill than to dig out the underlying causes of ill health. It's always simpler to say, "Oh, well, it's just old age," than to help patients change their lifestyle.

The point is, doctors are only human. When we ascribe super-human capabilities to them, blindly accept every word they say as gospel, and fail to take responsibility for our own health, we set ourselves on a course for premature "old age," disability and potential disaster.

Living and Learning

Another point I want to make at the very beginning of this book is that I'm not a doctor or a medical researcher. I'm not a scientist or a sociologist or any other kind of "expert" on longevity. I don't have an M.D. or Ph.D. degree. The fact is, my formal education ended in my early teens when I quit school and left home to make my way on my own. But in a sense, that was the beginning of my real education – a practical, common-sense learning experience that continues to this day.

In the nearly 50 years since then, I've never stopped learning. My life represents a constant and ongoing process of self-education. I believe nature equipped me with remarkable instincts for maintaining a healthy lifestyle. But I haven't been content to rely only on those instincts. I've also learned by reading, listening, observing, experimenting and discovering what works to improve my own body and mind, as well as the bodies and minds of those close to me and those thousands I've trained. Throughout a diversified career as a bodybuilder, a world-champion professional wrestler, a pioneer of the health club industry, a real estate developer, a professional pilot and the operator of an aircraft service company, I've never stopped learning about physical, mental and psychological health.

I consider myself a sort of "walking laboratory." I've experienced first-hand what the age-retarding foods, supplements, exercises, drugs and medical/surgical procedures that I recommend can do for a person. I recently underwent surgery on both shoulders to correct nerve damage caused by old wrestling injuries. The speed with which my incisions healed and I achieved full recovery amazed the doctors – even those who had known me for a long time. But I wasn't surprised at all. I know what my body's capable of doing.

I can show you how to deal with the onslaughts of aging, too. I can show you how to stay healthier, heal faster and hold degenerative illnesses at bay. I can show you how to put more vigor and satisfaction in your life – more than you ever dreamed possible.

Aren't You Dead Yet?

Our government, meanwhile, is no ally in our quest for longer, fuller lives. On the contrary, our government is vitally concerned that not too many of us live too long beyond retirement age. The Social Security system has been in deep financial trouble for a long time. And as the bumper crop of "boomers" born between 1946 and 1955 approach the point where they stop paying into the system and start withdrawing from it, the situation becomes more and more critical. Without revolutionary changes in who gets how much, most economic experts say Social Security will be bankrupt and out of business in another 20 years. So to keep this leaky boat afloat, be sure and do your duty as an older American – drop dead!

That's an increasingly popular philosophy among the politicians and bureaucrats who have gutted Social Security. It isn't likely to win many votes among senior citizens, but if big government has its way, we'll all be pushing up daisies pretty soon anyway.

Yet this is the very same government that forces people into retirement, whether they want to retire or not. It fosters a marketplace where experience, proven loyalty and accumulated knowledge count for nothing. Finding a good job when you're in your 50s takes a minor miracle, and beyond your 50s, forget it! The government creates rules that degrade and discriminate against every older wage-earner. It encourages industry to put as many over-50 employees out to pasture as possible – and as quickly as possible. "Go on," it says, "hurry up and retire – and then hurry up and die."

Our national approach to retirement is stupid and paradoxical. It grows more impossible to justify – and pay for – every year.

Airline pilots, for example, are pushed into mandatory retirement when they turn 60, although a lot of 60-year-old pilots are actually healthier and in better condition than some of their counterparts in their 30s and 40s. This is a travesty. Health, not age, should determine our ability to hold a job.

And while this travesty goes on, the fact remains that millions of Americans can't afford to retire at 65, much less at 60. Many people have no choice but to continue working if they expect to pay their bills. Millions more will be confronted with this situation as the baby boom generation nears traditional retirement age. A sizable percentage of the boomers will still be paying off their kids' education and/or facing mortgages on $250,000 homes when they reach 65. How are they going to survive on $800 a month in Social Security benefits?

Regardless of what happens to the Social Security system in the next few years, more and more Americans are going to find they have no option but to continue working beyond age 65 to maintain the lifestyle they want. Within the next decade or two, it will become standard procedure for wage-earners to stay on the job to age 70 or 75 or even 80.

If you're among these workers with heavy and continuing financial obligations, you have a tremendous need to maintain your health and vigor. You'll have to protect yourself more effectively than ever against the ravages associated with advancing age. Otherwise, you'll be courting disaster.

This, in turn, will put more pressure on the workplace to find more jobs for older employees. Age discrimination could become even more punitive and widespread.

Incidentally, the failing Social Security system isn't the only governmental adversary of the over-50 citizen. The FDA is another power-mad federal agency that does its best to keep American consumers from obtaining potentially beneficial drugs that are perfectly legal in most other countries. The FDA tries to control every product related in any way to health or nutrition – and it usually succeeds. We'll talk a lot more about how to circumvent the tyranny of the FDA later.

Don't Cheat Yourself

There's only one way to thwart these plotters. Beginning today, all of us past 50 have to start changing our own thinking about aging. We have to begin taking responsibility for our own lives, our own health, our own happiness and well being. We have to stop letting our system and our society relegate us to second-class status and deliberately destructive treatment just because we've passed a certain birthday.

As over-50 Americans, what you and I have to understand is that the conspiracy can't succeed without our cooperation. And millions of us are cooperating with it, although we may not realize it. We're unwittingly cooperating because we've been conditioned to cooperate and do what's expected of us by others. We accept the idea that our bodies and minds have to start unraveling and falling apart. We accept the idea that we aren't strong enough or alert enough to do the things we used to do. We accept the idea that we aren't much good for anything except dozing in front of the TV, taking our medicine and slowing turning into a mass of wrinkles, blubber and dead brain cells.

We're letting ourselves be "psyched out." We're being sold a bill of goods, and we're buying it. We're being fed a lot of BS, and we're swallowing it. When we do, we're cheating and short-changing ourselves.

If we refuse to get sick and die simply to enrich the "sickness industry," the conspiracy fails. If we refuse to stop working and thinking and contributing and creating (and, yes, maybe even procreating) just because we've reached age 55 or 60 or 65, the conspiracy can't succeed. If we stay vital and busy and productive, and refuse to accept the negative judgments of "the system," we can not only surprise society; we can also surprise ourselves. If we hold onto our health, our vigor, our faculties, our looks, our dignity and our independence, the plotters won't have a prayer.

And we can do it!

Accept the Challenge

Aging is a challenge, but it doesn't have to be a one-way ticket to limbo. The advancing years can be an adventure, not an ordeal. It's up to each of us whether to meet the challenge or dodge it. If you want to sit on the porch and rock, fine. But if you want to rock around the clock, you ought to be able to do that, too. After all, you've paid your dues. Aging offers us unique opportunities, if we're willing to explore them. The old saying that "you're not getting older; you're getting better" is a whole lot more than just empty words.

That statement is truer today than ever before. We have the knowledge, science, technology, tools and products to make it true. It can come true for you, starting right now. You can stand up and fight the aging conspiracy. You can disprove once and for all the phony idea that only physical and mental disability, defeat, deterioration and slow death await us after age 50 or 60.

This idea is as outmoded today as the Model T and the "Flying Jenny." But there was a time when it was solidly supported by fact. A century or two ago, most people wore themselves out long before their time with long hours of tedious, backbreaking physical labor. The typical wage-earner worked 60 or 70 hours a week for a survival-level income. People paid little attention to what they ate. As long as food was filling and affordable, nothing else mattered.

Meanwhile, infectious, highly contagious diseases such as

smallpox, tuberculosis, diphtheria, typhoid and influenza cut down millions in the prime of life and trimmed many years off the average life expectancy. Only a small minority of working-class people ever made it to the "retirement age" of 65. The rest died before they reached that milestone.

Those few who could afford a life of leisure and plenty often killed themselves through destructive habits and over-indulgence. And even the world's wealthiest individuals couldn't buy the phenomenal products and services we enjoy in the 1990s, much less the overall quality of life that the average American takes for granted.

A Whole New Ballgame

But that was in the distant past. Today, an ever-increasing percentage of people not only reach age 65, but age 85 and 95 and 105. One in eight Americans is now 65 or older. By 2030, that figure will climb to one in five. A baby born in 2000 – just five years from now – will have a life expectancy of nearly 80 years at birth. At some point in the next century, the median age of the U.S. population is expected to climb to 50. That means there will be as many people over 50 as there are under 50.

Incredible!

And the trends that will take us to that point are already in motion. Right now – today – we've got a whole new ballgame when it comes to age and aging. Are you ready to play that game? Are you ready to win it?

Just think about it for a moment: What would it be like if, instead of viewing age 50 as a time to "start slowing down and taking it easy," to start "planning for retirement," or even as the "beginning of the end," we saw it as what it actually should be – the beginning of the second half of life? What if people took it for granted that there were as many good times still ahead of them at 50 as there were behind them?

Would they still be ready to retire at 60 or 62 or 65? Would they be willing to spend the last 35 to 40 years of their lives knitting and whittling? I doubt it!

Are you ready for "prime time"? Are you ready for your second 50 years? Are you ready to make that "second 50" the most enjoyable, triumphant part of your life?

Shooting for 150

If what I'm saying sounds exaggerated, just take a look at the cold, hard statistics in population trends – and what the experts project will happen over the next few decades:

• The fastest growing segment of the population in the United States and other industrialized nations is the 85-and-older age group. Between 1960 and 1990, the overall U.S. population grew 39 percent, but the ranks of those 85 and older jumped by an incredible 232 percent.

• Today, there are already about 250,000 Americans over 100 years old. But by the year 2040, some population demographers predict that number will soar to 4 million or more. Personally, I think that's just the beginning. By the end of the next century, living to be 100 is likely to be as commonplace as living to 75 is today.

According to the Guinness Book of World Records, the world's oldest living person in 1995 is Jeanne Calment of Arles, France. Jeanne's 120 years old, and one doctor calls her the "Michael Jordan of aging." But a century from now, Jeanne's age group is likely to be so crowded nobody will even give a 120-year-old a second thought. With the advance of science, technology and human understanding of the factors that cause the body and mind to age, I firmly believe we will see some hardy people living to 150 – maybe even more – by the late 21st century.

This is no pipedream, friends. The time has come when anyone who takes care of himself or herself and follows a simple set of guidelines can expect to live to be 100. There's no guarantee, of course, that all of us will actually realize this expectation. We may be lost at sea trying to swim the English Channel at age 80, or fatally hurt in a skiing accident on our 90th birthday, or shot by a jealous husband (or wife) at age 95. But that's no reason not to expect the best and most of our "second 50."

Be the Best You Can Be

That "second 50" is within the grasp of anyone willing to reach out for it. I'm convinced of that. I've devoted nearly a half-century of personal research to the goal of enhancing my own health, strength, vitality, appearance, sexuality – and longevity. My wife, Clare, and I have shown thousands of men and women of all ages the way to better bodies, better looks, more stamina and a richer, fuller life.

In this process, we've pioneered many new concepts related to staying healthy, fit and youthful.

When I was 13 years old, I set out to maximize the assets nature had given me and minimize the liabilities. One of those assets was a burning ambition to be the best I could possibly be. Another was an in-born instinct that told me what was self-defeating and destructive to the human body, mind and spirit. I knew inherently, for instance, that smoking cigarettes was wrong.

Even as a teenager, I could tell that smoking inflicted harm on the body that no amount of exercise or nutrition could offset. That was long before there were warning labels on cigarette packages, long before the American Heart Association, the American Cancer Society and the U.S. surgeon general condemned smoking. People laughed when I told them smoking was unhealthy, but I knew I was right about smoking, and my instincts eventually turned out to be accurate. Today, smoking is universally recognized among medical experts as the number one preventable cause of death in the country.

Common-Sense "Secrets"

I also developed a strong belief in bodybuilding at a time when it was frowned on and ridiculed by practically all professional athletes, trainers and medical people. I used it to build the physical strength and endurance that made me one of the world's top pro wrestlers in a career that spanned 20 years and 5,000 professional bouts. Today, of course, virtually every training program in college and professional sports includes weight-resistance exercises. And even such renowned medical authorities as Dr. Kenneth Cooper, founder of the world-famous Cooper Clinic and the "father of aerobics," now recognize the benefits of weight training.

In some cases, it's taken 50 years for some of my theories and ideas to be substantiated and widely accepted, but the secrets I've learned along the way aren't really "secrets" at all. They're the products of common sense, experience, a willingness to work and learn, a bit of experimentation – and self-discipline. It's my firm belief that nothing worthwhile in this life can be accomplished without self-discipline. How much of this you have will definitely affect your lifestyle and lifespan. If you can exercise self-discipline, the steps to a healthier, longer life are simple. They're steps anyone can master – if he or she wants to. And the whole purpose of this book is to share them with you.

Even if you don't think of yourself as a person with a lot of self-control, the good results you can see in yourself after just a few weeks of putting the principles of this book into practice in your life will serve to strengthen your resolve. The natural "high" that comes from feeling good about yourself will give you willpower you never knew you possessed.

A Treatable Disease

I'm 62 years old, but I'm planning for another 40 to 50 years of healthy, active, exciting life. I fully expect to be doing just about everything I'm doing today 25 or 30 or 40 years from now. You can do the same.

If you're interested in staying young, vital, attractive and sexy during your second 50 years, here's my message to you in a nutshell:

The degenerative process that we know as aging is simply another treatable disease – with the emphasis on the word *treatable*. Today, we have at our disposal all the tools necessary to hold this disease at bay, often for decades. It's something we all have to live with and reckon with as we move beyond age 50, but effective treatments are readily available to anyone who wants them.

If you were suffering from a severe infection, would you choose to take antibiotics to eliminate it, or would you choose to let it kill you? In my view, the reasonable, intelligent course would be to treat it with antibiotics. The same identical situation exists with aging. Will you control it with the amazing new foods, age-defeating exercises and other "wonder drugs" now available, or will you succumb to it long before your time?

The answer, of course, is up to you.

That "Old" Feeling

Our specific chronological age is much less important than our physical condition and psychological state. You can "get old" at any point in life. Believe me, I know people in their 30s and 40s who are "older" than I am in every respect except for the number of years they've lived.

"Getting old" is one of the most terrible, insidious diseases I can think of. In a way, it's even worse than such mass killers as heart disease and cancer, because there's so often no real reason for it to happen. It feeds on bad habits and self-abusive behavior. It proliferates in the face of negativism, stress, frustration and low self-esteem. It grows more severe each time we look in the mirror and hate what we see, each time we try to deny the reading on the bathroom scales, each time we say something to ourselves like, "What difference does it make how I look? I'm so old and fat nobody cares anyway."

All of us get down at times, but that has nothing to do with aging. In fact, teenagers and young adults probably have just as many feelings of gloom and doom as we over-50s do. But when you reach the point that you don't care enough about yourself to look your best, when it's no longer important to you to be attractive to the opposite sex, then you're giving in to the disease of aging. You're getting old in the worst, most destructive sense of the term. I don't intend to let that happen to me, and you shouldn't, either.

No matter what other people – including your doctor – may tell you, it is not inevitable that you lose your sex appeal, your sex drive or your sense of wellbeing just because the birthdays are piling up. Feeling attractive and sexy is one of the main manifestations of health and vitality.

It's Never Too Late

There is no cut-off age for attractiveness and sexuality. Mae West, Gloria Swanson and Marlene Dietrich were glamorous film stars well into their 70s. At 75, my friend and fellow bodybuilder, Bob Delmonteque, is still a "hunk" who can turn many a younger woman's head. At 73, my friend and mentor, Joe Weider, one of the true pioneers of physical fitness in this country, has more strength, endurance and vitality than most guys half his age. Any number of men have fathered children in their 70s.

Because of the strides in science and technology, there's never been less reason to "act your age" than there is today. George Foreman is a world heavyweight boxing champion at age 45. Several major league baseball players are in their 40s. Bob Hope is still cracking jokes at 92. George Burns is planning his 100th birthday party in Las Vegas.

Remember this: Regardless of your chronological age,

you're never too old to look and feel younger or reach out for new vitality. And despite your chronological age, your biological and psychological age can be much younger. As long as you're breathing, it's never too late to strive for satisfaction or dare to improve yourself.

Combatting all the symptoms of aging – the physical, the emotional and the psychological – is what this book is all about. I'm going to show you how to meet the challenge of aging in every phase of your life. I'm going to show you how the right combination of diet, exercise, nutritional supplements, remarkable new drugs and products, new scientific techniques and common-sense changes in your lifestyle can stop the deterioration we associate with aging before it starts. I'm going to tell you in simple, straightforward terms how you can look, feel and perform better at 75 – or 85 or more – than many people do at 35.

I'm also going to give you some powerful ammunition to fight the conspiracy against over-50 Americans and counteract the unfair age discrimination directed at us by our society and our system. I'm going to show you how to keep your self-esteem, your sex appeal, your zest for life, your fighting spirit. To paraphrase an old song, I'm going to show you how to "accentuate the positive" and "eliminate the negative."

In short, I'm going to prove to you that the second 50 years of your life can be even more fulfilling, satisfying and rewarding than the first 50!

"To be seventy years young is sometimes far more cheerful and hopeful than to be forty years old."
—OLIVER WENDELL HOLMES

CHAPTER
2

The Psychology of Staying Young

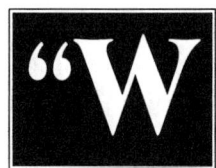hy do I feel so depressed and hopeless?"

"Why am I always so tired and worn-out?"

"How much longer can I stand the stress of this rat race? Is it really worth it?"

Almost all of us ask ourselves questions like these. But often we tell ourselves there aren't really any definitive answers. We try to shrug off the feelings of inadequacy, frustration, pessimism and defeat that trigger the questions.

"That's the way life is," we say. "There's nothing I can do about it."

"Everybody feels that way," we rationalize, "so it must be normal."

And millions of us eventually come to the same convenient conclusion:

"I guess I'm just getting old!"

We may pass it off as a bitter joke, but there's nothing funny about it. And we definitely aren't laughing when we say it. What we're doing is admitting – both to the rest of the world and to ourselves – that we don't have the energy, stamina or mental alertness we want to have. We don't feel as vigorous or virile as we'd like to feel. We don't bear up as well under pressure as we did at other times. It seems harder to cope with the physical and psychological demands of life.

It's easy to blame it all on age – too easy. And all too often, our friends, relatives, acquaintances and co-workers are ready and willing to reinforce that idea.

"You know, you're not getting any younger," they say. "Maybe you should slow down a little."

I say "baloney!" If you accept this wrongheaded notion as fact, it can make you old long before your time. It can rob you of your natural vitality. It can make you first complacent, then comatose. It's already done that to untold millions of people. So I say let's do our best to stamp it out right now.

Don't Be Brainwashed

This distressingly prevalent "logic" is a prime example of how we let ourselves be brainwashed into giving up the rewards, pleasures and challenges of life because we're getting older. Look at it this way: A ten-year-old kid isn't as young as he used to be, either. But he ought to be stronger, smarter, more mature, more experienced and better able to deal with life than he was when he was in diapers.

The same is true for people over 50. If you have a fit body, a healthy lifestyle and a positive attitude, there's absolutely no reason to be any less energetic, less active, less productive or less enthusiastic about life when you're 60, 70 or 80 than you were when you were 25 or 30. There's no reason to be less fulfilled, either. You don't have to walk slower or quit riding a bicycle. You don't have to give up skiing or make love less often. You don't have to stop caring how you look or striving for success. You don't have to stop planning your next big adventure – whether it's a romantic conquest, starting a new business or setting sail for Tahiti in a 50-foot boat.

Anyone who tells you different has to be classified as one of the negative forces that confront us every day. These are forces that all of us must either overcome and defeat or somehow learn to ignore. Otherwise, they'll defeat us. They may even make us sick. And carried to their ultimate extreme, they could actually kill us.

A Negative Environment

Here in this land of unparalleled wealth, accomplishment and promise, we live in an atmosphere of terrible, debilitating negativism. Every day of our lives, we are bombarded from all directions by destructive negative forces. Think about it:

For many of us, the onslaught begins when we open our morning newspapers. There, staring back at us from the printed pages, are endless tales of horror, calamity and woe. Crime in the streets. Famine in Africa. Violence in the Middle East. Death on the highway. Mindless wars that go on and on without cause or reason. Our cities are crumbling. Killer diseases are running rampant with no cure in sight. Taxes are going up and there's still no money to fix what's wrong. Our lawmakers do nothing but steal from the public and squabble among themselves. All politicians are crooks. Unemployment is climbing. The economy's getting worse. Our schools are falling apart. Our teenagers are hooked on drugs. Our kids are out of control. It goes on and on and on.

In the evenings, we come home from work and get another dose or two of the same gloom-and-doom on the TV newscasts. Even the occasional positive stories all seem to have a negative twist. The media plans it that way. It's called "objective journalism."

Is it any wonder we creep off to bed practically humming with negative vibes?

Is Anything All Right?

And how about some of the people we encounter as we go through our daily rounds? It seems that every place of employment has its share of perpetual malcontents and chronic complainers. Aren't these guys a joy and a pleasure to work with? Doesn't their bright-eyed, upbeat approach make you love to be around them?

For God's sake, don't make the mistake of asking one of them "How are you?" He just might tell you:

"Oh, I've got this terrible cold. And there's this terrible pain in my back. And the baby kept me up all night crying. And my wife's ticked off about something. And I'll never get through with all this work on my desk. And my car has to have a new engine. And I'm so broke I don't see how I'll make it till payday. And the boss is always picking on me. And I hate this job. And

my house is falling down. And my shoes hurt my feet. And . . . "
And after a while, you want to run off screaming.

Negativism is highly contagious, you see. It spreads like an epidemic. Have you ever noticed how one "carrier" can infect a whole roomful of people in a matter of minutes? Misery loves company, and pretty soon, everybody's bitching and complaining about something. Keeping a positive outlook in an atmosphere like this is one of the hardest things in the world to do.

In our society, growing old could be called the "ultimate negative." But how could anyone who lives or works in this kind of atmosphere help but feel old and grumpy and frazzled?

Make Your Escape

So what do you do about it? Nobody can avoid all the negative influences in our world. But there are ways to minimize them in your life – simple ways that don't involve quitting your job, becoming a hermit, moving to a desert island, or even kicking in the screen of your TV.

If the 10 o'clock news worries or distresses you, turn it off. If the front page of your newspaper gets you down, read the comics, the sports or "Dear Abby" instead. Hang up on telephone solicitors who want to tell you how much you need burial insurance or a cemetery plot. Avoid people who like to carp incessantly about how the world, the country, the state, the city and the neighborhood are going to hell in a handbasket.

Anytime a conversation turns into too much of a "downer," I try to change the subject. If that doesn't work, I simply excuse myself and walk away. Then I look for somebody to talk to who can be halfway cheerful.

If I feel discomfort, or even pain, I don't burden other people with it. You shouldn't, either. In the first place, very few people really give a damn how you or I feel, anyway. And talking about it doesn't relieve the pain or discomfort; if anything it only makes it worse.

If you wake up in the morning feeling terrible, it won't do the slightest bit of good to say out loud, "Jeez, I feel terrible." I guarantee it won't. Maybe you can't be totally rah-rah positive under such circumstances, but verbalizing your bad feelings only makes you concentrate on them more fully. Instead, you could try saying, "Oh, well, I'll feel better later." If you can't manage that, just grin at yourself in the mirror and don't say anything.

The power of suggestion is stronger than many people realize. Tell yourself you feel bad often enough, and you will feel bad. Tell yourself how tired you are 50 times a day, and chances are, you'll barely have the energy to fall into bed when you get home in the evening. There's no way to calculate the number of psychologically induced illnesses that send Americans to doctors and hospitals each year, but it's safe to say they run into the millions. These are so-called "psychosomatic" disorders with no physical basis whatsoever.

Psychological factors can affect your blood pressure, your heart rate, your respiration, your temperature – virtually all your vital signs. They can trigger asthma, insomnia, vertigo, headaches, nausea, diarrhea, constipation, palpitations, rashes, gout and God-knows-what-else. Doctors generally agree that the vast majority of cases of male impotence are psychologically based with no discernible physical cause.

On the other hand, if you tell yourself you feel good, you just may. And if your message to yourself is effective enough, it may not only spare you many days of "feeling bad" but also help shield you from actual physical illness. When you do get sick, a positive psyche can speed your recovery, or even allow you to survive indefinitely with an illness that would quickly prove fatal to many other people.

One of the things that amazes me is that people who would seem to have the most legitimate reasons for feeling miserable are often more cheerful than the rest of us. I know a man who was diagnosed with terminal cancer four or five years ago. Yet whenever I call him on the phone and ask how he's doing, his reply is always the same.

"Tremendous!" he'll say. "Fabulous!"

I have no doubt that his positive, upbeat attitude has lengthened his life, and I hope it continues to do so.

Join a New Circle

If you want to break out of the trap of negativism, it's important to try to pinpoint the sources. Only then can we begin to systematically eliminate them or minimize their ill effects.

Who are the friends and co-workers you spend time with during lunch hours and breaks? Who are the members of your carpool or bridge club or bowling team? Who do you stop off with for a drink after work? Are they all in your same age bracket – maybe even older? What do they talk about?

If you surround yourself with people who focus constantly on the down side of life, their opinions and values will inevitably rub off on you. Lunch and break conversations that are dominated by talk about retirement, chronic ailments, recent funerals, financial problems, marital unhappiness and who's dying of what can be real bummers. They can not only get on your nerves and upset your digestion; they can also bog you down in serious depression and despair. Warning: This kind of talk may be hazardous to your health.

On the other hand, the optimism and enthusiasm of others can also be contagious. In our cynical world, it may not be as easy to spread cheer as it is to spread misery, but when we encounter someone with a genuinely sunny outlook, it's hard not to feel a little lift.

A lot of us subject ourselves to continuous, destructive negativism without consciously realizing what we're doing or that we can find positive alternatives if we look for them. If this is happening to you, maybe you should consider joining a new carpool or finding a new circle of lunchtime and after-work companions.

Instead of sticking with your contemporaries in the over-50 set, why not find a place for yourself in a younger group – people, say, in their 20s and 30s? You may be amazed at the difference in the way they talk, act and think. Chances are, their whole approach to life is different from your former circle. And you may be amazed at the difference they can cause in you.

Suddenly, you're not hearing about death, disease, disability and doom at every turn. Instead, you're hearing your tablemates discussing their latest romances, their new cars, their favorite sports, the hot new movie they saw last night, the exciting weekend trip they have coming up, their plans and dreams for the future. What a refreshing change!

Don't "Date" Yourself

One thing I like about younger people is their attitude toward age – which, in most cases, is no attitude at all. They simply don't think about it that much. They're too busy living for this day, this moment. And it might surprise you how many people in their 20s can't tell by looking whether you're 38 or 61. What's more, they don't really care. Age is still relatively unimportant to them. They haven't become obsessed with it the way so many over-50 men and women are. Their whole lives are before them.

And just because you're older and wiser and more savvy to the ways of the world than they are, that doesn't mean you can't learn some valuable lessons from them.

This is one reason I try never to age-relate myself. I try not to talk about the "good old days," and I studiously avoid such expressions as "when I was your age" or "when you're as old as I am." To me, nothing brands you more quickly as a member of the "older generation." Remember, you're only as old as you feel, think, act and talk – so don't "date" yourself unnecessarily.

Just as the gloomy, dreary patterns of thought and speech associated with "getting old" tend to rub off on those exposed to them, so do the high hopes, excitement and positive outlook of youth.

"I Forget How Old I Am"

This is one reason that so many widowed or divorced men in their 50s, 60s, 70s and 80s (and an increasing number of women in this age group, too) are drawn to much younger mates. Sure, part of it is pure physical attraction to the "bloom of youth." But maybe even more important is the psychological boost you get from being with someone who's still enjoying life instead of withdrawing from it. Someone who's living each day with relish instead of counting the days to retirement. Someone who's looking ahead instead of mourning the passage of the "good old days."

"I feel more like I'm 38 than 58," one friend of mine says. "One reason is because I married a woman who's 20 years younger than I am. She likes to go out and have a good time, and she keeps me busy doing fun stuff. But another reason is because all our close friends are now in her age group, not mine. I tend to identify with these younger people and their approach to life. Most of my old acquaintances don't do anything these days but sit around groaning and complaining. It makes me feel bad to be around them. I don't even think of myself as being one of those old fogies anymore. Frankly, I forget a lot of the time how old in years I really am."

This friend's experience is becoming more and more commonplace. I know any number of men who married much younger women and started second families in their late 40s and early to mid-50s. Now they're shopping for larger and more expensive homes, planning family trips to Disney World, and coaching their kids' soccer teams at an age when many of their contemporaries are sinking quietly into an old-age mentality and the "long nap" of retirement.

I'm certainly not suggesting that everyone should dump his or her longtime mate and go in search of a "new model." But I also know of many marriages in which one spouse has grown far older than the other in a psychological sense, even though they're both very close together in chronological age. When you feel young psychologically, it only stands to reason that you look and act young, too. You pay more attention to appearance, fitness and sex appeal.

Regardless of how long they've been together, when two people find themselves traveling in different directions, compatibility may no longer be possible. Romantic feelings between them may be totally snuffed out as the gap widens. In cases like this, unless one partner is willing to change or both can somehow compromise, it may be better for them to go their separate ways.

Tuning in to Youth

Maybe you aren't interested in pursuing younger women – or younger men. Maybe you don't want to go out dancing every night, or whirl through life on a merry-go-round. Maybe you don't want to go on a camping trip every weekend or spend every weekend in Vegas, either. Maybe you're not into kid games or taking on huge mortgages. Maybe you have no desire to drive a sports car or party until the wee hours. But the point is, almost anyone can find ways to tune in to a more youthful wavelength, at least once in a while.

I know a university professor, for example, who makes far more money in another professional field and has no real financial need to keep teaching. But he stays on because, as he puts it: "Being in a roomful of 20-year-olds is exhilarating. It keeps me in touch with what the next generation of movers and shakers is saying and doing. I think it helps to keep me young."

I think so, too. So my suggestion to any over-50 individual is this: Take stock of the people you spend most of your time with. If all of them are in your same age bracket, or even older, it's not a good sign. Cultivating a few friendships with younger people could do wonders for your state of mind and your outlook on life.

And don't think you'll be boring or imposing on your younger friends. I honestly believe that most men and women in their 20s and 30s value friendships with more mature, more experienced people. (Notice I didn't say "older.") They can benefit from our accumulated knowledge and wisdom just as we can benefit from their freshness and vitality.

Reward or Death Sentence?

Let's go back to the subject of retirement for a few minutes. Let's examine the whole concept of "hanging 'em up" at a certain point in life and taking it easy from that point on. Let's look at how that concept originated, how it grew, and how it has become so deeply ingrained in the consciousness of our society. Let's look at the psychological impact it has on every working person. Let's look at the fallacies that underlie it.

For a few fortunate people, retirement turns out to be exactly what they hoped it would be – a refreshing, relaxing reward for decades of hard work, yet a busy, productive, satisfying experience as well. For countless others, it quickly deteriorates into tedium and a sense of worthlessness, aggravated by severe – often unexpected – financial pressures. It can become a lingering misery of want, uncertainty, loneliness and fear. But at its worst extremes, it literally becomes a death sentence.

All of us have heard stories about someone who retired in apparent good health, only to drop dead a short time later. One of the most widely publicized examples of such a tragedy was the legendary college football coach, Paul "Bear" Bryant. When Bryant stepped down as head coach at the University of Alabama and was no longer able to plot strategy on the sidelines or urge his beloved Crimson Tide to victory, life for him was simply no longer worth living. Within a few months, he was dead.

Undoubtedly, the same thing happens to tens of thousands of lesser-known retirees every year. So often, a person's work is literally his whole life, his whole reason for being here. Without it, he or she has no identity. For someone like this, retirement is the end. Nothing is left.

The Secret of Survival

Others, of course, not only survive for decades in retirement, but actually thrive. Some of those who fare best as retirees will tell you candidly it's because they're basically lazy. They enjoy doing nothing, having no responsibilities to meet, no orders to follow, no schedules to keep. They're the same kind of people who never let a "sick day" go to waste during their working years. You know, the ones who always take an extra five minutes to get back to their desks or workbenches after breaks, who can stretch a trip to the water fountain to 10 minutes and a trip to the restroom to 20. They're always among the last to arrive in the morning and first out the door at the end of the day. And they always prefer "comp time" to overtime.

They're the kind of folks who can spend a whole day fishing and never get a single bite. Actually, you get the feeling they'd rather be "just drowning worms" than be distracted by something tugging on their line.

For people like this, retirement is the ultimate opportunity to screw off. Being paid not to work has been their goal in life from the beginning, and now they've achieved that goal permanently. There may not be any statistics to support me, but I know deep down inside that this type of individual probably lives longer in retirement than anybody else. If he dies, he won't be getting something for nothing anymore, and that's motivation enough to keep him breathing.

The rest of us, however, just aren't built that way. We may have a little larceny in our hearts, but we don't – we can't – carry it to such extremes. To us, productivity, a sense of accomplishment and self-worth and the ability to take care of ourselves are the very essence of life. So if we expect to survive very long in retirement, we have to figure out a way to hang onto these attributes.

The people I know who have made the best adjustment to retirement are those who, if anything, are busier today and more engrossed in what they're doing than they were when they were "working." If retirement represents a mere change in direction, rather than a dead end, it can be a truly positive experience. If you're an auto mechanic who's always dreamed of being a hunting guide or an insuranceman whose real love is making violins, and retirement gives you the chance to realize that dream or fulfill that love, it can be one of the best times of life.

Otherwise, regardless of what everyone else expects or what you've been led to believe, you might be well-advised to keep right on working for another 20 or 30 years.

It Started With FDR

What is this thing called retirement, anyway? Where did we get the idea that everything has to come to a screeching halt when we turn 65 (or, in many cases, earlier)? The idea of retirement has become an integral part of our national philosophy in the 60 years since the Social Security Act of 1935 became the law of the land.

Until the administration of President Franklin D. Roosevelt instituted Social Security, there was no set age for retirement. And since there were no automatic government benefits for retirees, except for some small pension payments to a select few, most people worked as long as they were able.

At the time, the average life expectancy in the United States was just a shade over 60 years, so the average person didn't give much thought to retirement at 65. Only the "unaverage" lived that long. And although many people were forced by ill health to stop working well before their 65th birthdays, it also wasn't uncommon for people whose health and stamina permitted to stay on the job until they were well into their 70s or 80s.

Something else about Social Security as it was originally conceived: It was never intended to serve as the sole support of retirees and their mates. It was designed to help bridge the gap between what people needed to live and what they could save on their own plus whatever assistance they could get from other sources. Social Security was never envisioned as the end-all, be-all that millions of people consider it today.

One key reason that the Social Security System is on the verge of bankruptcy is because the politicians and bureaucrats have conveniently forgotten that fact. Over the past 40 or so years, they've tried to make Social Security keep pace with the cost of living. They've failed, but in the process, they've instilled the idea in the public that a "free ride" awaits us after we turn 65, courtesy of the federal government.

Don't Outlive Your Car

But the "ride" can be a rough one for anybody who tries to live on the $800 or less per month that the typical Social Security recipient draws. Certainly no one with an unpaid mortgage on his home can survive on that amount alone. Neither can anyone who lives in rented housing, or anyone who still has children in school, or anyone with car payments, charge account debts or any sort of extra obligations over and above the basics.

Most of the time, Social Security provides about enough for an individual or couple to buy clothes, groceries and gasoline and pay local taxes and utility bills. There's usually little or nothing left for home maintenance, car repairs, insurance, household furnishings, medicine and other essentials – much less such "luxuries" as travel, recreation, entertaining, gifts, cosmetics, hair care, church or charitable contributions, laundry and dry cleaning, etc. In fact, an increasing number of Social Security recipients have to rely on food stamps to have enough to eat.

If your car wears out and you have to buy another one, where does the money come from? If your roof leaks and your plumbing's worn out, how do you pay for fixing it? You don't – not on Social Security. You're not supposed to outlive your car or your roof or your plumbing, remember?

Is This What We Work For?

And what makes matters so much worse is that, under federal regulations, you aren't allowed to earn more than $7,000 or $8,000 per year in additional income. If you do, Uncle Sam cuts your Social Security benefits accordingly. You can have an income of $1 million a year or more from investments and/or interest, and that's OK. It's only earned income that's restricted. Why? To keep you out of the job market, of course. That's the whole idea of the earned income restriction.

Is this the kind of retirement all of us should be eagerly looking forward to? Is a subsistence-level existence on less than $10,000 per year – or no more than $17,000 or $18,000 at the very most – supposed to be our reward for working 40-plus years? Is this the reason we pay those hefty Social Security taxes every payday – taxes that we're given no choice about paying?

I don't think so. I can't imagine anything more depressing. And I frankly can't see how a retiree's life could be anything but dreary and wretched under circumstances like these.

There is a loophole in this punitive system, however. If you can manage to stay on the job for just five additional years –

until you turn 70 – then you can not only draw increased Social Security benefits but do so with no restrictions on the amount of additional income you can earn. It amazes me how many people are approaching traditional retirement age without knowing this.

The Choice Is Yours

If you're not one of the unfortunate thousands who are pushed out to pasture involuntarily at 60 or 65, you do have a choice You have the choice of working longer and giving yourself additional income – both before and after retirement – plus valuable extra earning time to achieve financial security for your real old age.

In years to come, I have no doubt that millions and millions of Americans will choose this option.

In the meantime, though, we continue to be subjected to intense psychological pressure – brainwashing, if you will – to retire at the "normal" age. We continue to be subtly "conditioned" to the idea that, beyond 60 or 65, we are no longer able to be productive, performing members of the workforce.

Unfortunately, many Americans are in fragile health by the time they reach their 60s. But the reason most of them are is because they accepted "getting old" as an inevitability when they were in their 40s and 50s, and they didn't do what they needed to do to keep their minds and bodies fit and active and youthful. These people probably should retire, but there are millions and millions of others for whom retirement makes no sense at all.

If you're a healthy, capable man or woman in your 60s, 70s, 80s or even 90s, there's no reason to stop pursuing a career, earning money, achieving goals and building self-esteem until you actually want to stop. You are the only one who should be allowed to decide this. Nobody should have the right to make that decision for you – not corporate America, not the federal government, not the negative media, not the insurance companies, not the social planners, not society at large. Nobody!

And the sooner we realize that those of us over 50 have been targeted for psychological warfare by all these forces, the sooner we can defeat this tyranny.

Beware of the "Big Lie"

Adolf Hitler was a master at the psychology of the "big lie." He brainwashed an entire nation into following him blindly and unquestioningly to disaster. The technique was simple: Repeat something often enough, and no matter how outlandishly false it may be, people will eventually believe it.

That's exactly what's happened over the past 60 years in our national attitudes about aging. While science, technology and expanding knowledge have put an incredible arsenal of weapons against aging within our grasp, we've let ourselves be hookwinked by the "big lie." This enormous falsehood says we have to bow out of our work, curtail our activities, stop seeking fulfillment and satisfaction, forsake our achievements, and accept a mediocre semi-life of retirement – all because we've reached a certain chronological age.

Within that same period, Americans in general have been transformed from a people with a confident, positive, "can-do" philosophy to a people assailed by self-doubt and defeatism. We've been conditioned to react negatively to almost everything, to duck responsibilities and hard decisions, to "let the government do it," even when we know they're going to do it wrong.

But it's not too late to expose the "big lie" for what it is. It's not too late to take charge of your own destiny. It's not too late to think and act positively, to harness the amazing psychological powers that each of us possesses.

Your life isn't all behind you just because you're over 50. A vast, enticing chunk of it can still be ahead of you.

All you have to do is reach for it!

"I am an optimist. It doesn't seem much use being anything else."
—WINSTON CHURCHILL

CHAPTER 3

My Own Story – A Half-Century of Personal Research

My childhood can be summed up adequately in two words – precociousness and poverty. The dictionary defines that first term as "premature development of the mind and faculties," but, of course, I had no idea what it meant at the time. All I knew was that I didn't seem to think and react like other kids my age.

I knew exactly what it meant to be poor, though. My father worked as a welder, cab driver and at various other jobs where the pay was always meager and hours were always long. He called himself and his generation "the last of the Jewish workmen," and I guess they really were. Most Jews today are white-collar types.

I was born on January 12, 1933, in the Brownsville section of Brooklyn. If a historian were to pick the absolute lowest point of the Great Depression, that would almost certainly have been it. Times were as hard and as close to hopeless as they've ever been in this country. My parents, Sam and Kitty Bookbinder, named me Walter.

As a small boy, I lived in a dingy, roach-infested apartment that was cold in the winter, hot in the summer and generally miserable 12 months out of the year. There were eight of us crowded into three tiny bedrooms and one bath. My dad, my mother and I slept in one room. My Aunt Mary and her two kids stayed in another, and my grandparents occupied the third. Later on, my younger sister, Bobbie, came along, but by then we had a little more space. Can you imagine eight people having to share a single bathroom? We didn't have any major problems that I remember, but it left enough of an impression on me that I've always insisted on including a bathroom for each bedroom in every building I've ever had built.

One of the earliest things I can remember thinking as a kid was: "There's got to be something better in life than this!"

Call of the Wild World

In school, I was a loner. I didn't mingle with the other kids. I preferred losing myself in my own thoughts and daydreams. From the time I learned to read, I had a book in my hand almost constantly. I read everything I could get my hands on, from Jack London to Karl Marx. I especially liked London's classic, *The Call of the Wild*. The title seems prophetic as I look back on it today. By the time I was 10 or so, I could already hear the wide, wild world calling me.

The book that really changed my life, though, was one entitled *Martin Eden*. It was written as a novel, but it was actually Jack London's autobiography. The author told of running away from home and becoming an oyster pirate at the age of 13. I was enthralled with the adventures London wrote about. They made me more restless than ever, and more curious about the endless wonders that lay beyond the boundaries of my drab little domain. Right then, I started plotting my own escape.

Whenever I could scrape up the 10 cents it cost for admission, I went to the movies. Movies were even more exciting than books, because they visually portrayed an entire "other world" right there before your eyes. They depicted a life that was as enticing as it was foreign to me – fancy clothes, luxurious homes, flashy cars, beautiful women, dashing men, sophistication, wealth, power.

Although the movies were make-believe, I sensed that this "other world" was really out there. In New York, as in few other places on earth, immense wealth and dire poverty live within a few blocks of each other. Like every other poor kid from Brooklyn, I yearned for a share of what I saw on Fifth Avenue. But unlike many of the others, I was motivated to reach out and grasp it.

By the time of my 13th birthday, I knew I was soon going to leave home and strike out on my own. It wasn't that I didn't love my parents and family. It was just that I knew instinctively that, in order to succeed in life, I had to experience the world for myself – both the good and the bad it had to offer.

Developing a "Sixth Sense"

My first big adventure was triggered by my consuming interest in politics. I hitchhiked from Brooklyn all the way to Columbus, Ohio, for a major political convention. I was incredibly naive at the time. For example, I knew absolutely nothing about sex. My parents had never mentioned the subject, and since I always distanced myself from the other kids at school, I hadn't even picked up on most of the often-distorted "information" that adolescent boys usually exchange.

On my Ohio trip, I was given rides by some people who talked and acted very strangely. They made me extremely uncomfortable, and some "sixth sense" warned me not to have anything to do with them. These warnings steered me away from harm many times, along with an inherent understanding of right and wrong that I think every one of us carries around inside us.

This same "sixth sense" has served me well all my life. At a time when it seemed that almost every adult male smoked, and almost every teenage boy was tempted to start – and long before any medical warnings had been issued about smoking – it warned me that smoking was unhealthy and dangerous. As a result, I never touched a cigarette. I never experimented with illegal drugs, either.

Even at 13, I had enough sense to know I couldn't survive in the demanding, often hostile outside world without a plan, and I spent weeks formulating a pretty good one. Inspired by Jack London's adventures, I decided to go to sea.

I never gave much thought to trying to join the Navy, though. For one thing, the Navy had far more men than it needed at that time. World War II had been over for less than a year, and hundreds of thousands of sailors were being discharged and sent home. For another thing, I didn't want to be bound by the rigid military rules the Navy would impose on me. I didn't mind a reasonable amount of discipline, but at the same time, I wanted a freer, less restrictive way of life. I decided to join the merchant marine instead.

The merchant marine is a civilian organization supervised by the Coast Guard. To join, you must first be accepted by the union, then obtain your seaman's papers from the Coast Guard. The problem was, I was a good five years too young to qualify on either score. But I was big and husky for my age — I'd already started working out after reading some bodybuilding magazines — and, as I said, I had a plan.

A Lesson in Survival

It was simple, really. I had a friend named Paul Davis, who was six years older than I was and who agreed to let me borrow his birth certificate and identity. That was one obstacle out of the way. The next obstacle was raising some traveling money. That proved somewhat more difficult.

I tried working as a busboy in a restaurant, but I lasted only a few hours. Feeling the kind of desperation that only an impatient 13-year-old can feel, I did something that went against my very nature: I stole $12 from my grandmother. I vowed I'd pay her back with my first merchant marine paycheck. Then I bought a bus ticket to Norfolk, Virginia, a seaport town where I'd heard I could join the seafarers union.

To my bitter disappointment, the Norfolk union told me I was out of luck, that they weren't taking on any new men. Crestfallen, I headed back for New York, but decided to stop over in Baltimore to check out the situation there. I stumbled straight into a strike by the Sailors Union of the Pacific, and I impulsively volunteered to help walk the picket line. In return, when the strike was settled, some of the union members helped me get my seaman's papers.

It took two weeks for that to happen, though. And those two weeks were the toughest time of my young life. The round-trip bus fare from New York to Norfolk and back had taken most of my money. I was flat broke, and there was no way I could pay for lodging.

I spent my first night in Baltimore in a ratty all-night

striptease movie theatre. The place was full of derelicts and winos, and it reeked of urine and vomit. After that, I moved to the Greyhound bus station and spent the rest of the two weeks sleeping on a hard bench or on the waiting room floor, and washing up in the public restroom. Every night, the police came by and threatened to arrest me for vagrancy. But I still had my return ticket to New York and that gave me the right to stay at the depot. I was only a kid, but I was learning a valuable lesson in survival.

Meanwhile, the only money I had was a $2-a-day allowance from the union. I used most of it to buy milk to make sure I got enough protein to keep me going. Most kids my age would probably have spent their allowance on candy bars or potato chips, but I had read enough about nutrition to know better than that.

I also connived to get whatever free food I could. Once I saw a newspaper classified ad for hotdog vendors at a football game, and I rushed to the stadium. As soon as I was assigned a cart, I ate every last hotdog it contained, then left before anyone knew what I'd done.

When I was finally assigned to a ship after those two weeks, the first thing I did was make a beeline for the galley. I was too hungry to think straight, and I ate until I almost popped. And then, of course, when we put out to sea, I promptly got seasick. Today, I can look back on it as just another learning experience, but at the time, I thought I'd die for sure.

Years later, when I came back to Baltimore as a professional wrestler, I bought a new Cadillac there and drove down to the bus station for a nostalgic visit. I felt tears in my eyes as I looked out over the waiting room. In many ways, I no longer felt like the same person as the confused, homeless kid who had slept on the floor in one corner of the depot. But in another way, I never wanted to forget where I had come from and how hard life had been.

Home Again, Gone Again

My first fling as a seaman came to an early and ignoble end. Two buddies and I went ashore in a southern town. We got into an argument in a bar – an argument that quickly escalated into a brawl – and the next thing I knew, the bartender was coming at me with a butcher knife. In self-defense, I knocked him down.

But then I started kicking him, and that was a bad mistake. The three of us ended up in jail, charged with aggravated assault. When somebody told me I could get 10 years in prison for what I'd done, I responded like the overgrown child I was.

"But I'm only 13 years old," I pleaded. "Call my father and tell him to come get me out of here!"

Dad bailed me out, all right. To raise the money, he had to pawn the expensive camera I'd gotten for my bar mitzvah. He took me back to New York on a Friday. Three days later, I was on another ship and gone again. The call of the wild was just too strong for me to resist.

My parents didn't see me again for four long years.

By the time we were reunited, Walter, the immature boy who had run away at 13, no longer existed. In his place was a man who had traveled all over the globe and learned to make his way in a hard and unforgiving world. I'd discovered a lot about a lot of things, but the lessons I'd learned about sex and romance may have contributed more than anything else to the difference between the boy I had been and the man I now was.

My first encounter with sex had been an absolute disaster. It had been a brief, sweaty interlude in a filthy apartment with a gross, gum-smacking prostitute who looked far worse undressed than she did with her clothes on. For something I had anticipated so eagerly and for so long to turn into such a nightmare left me totally disgusted and disillusioned. Was this what guys were always talking about with such excitement? I couldn't believe it!

Soon, however, in a port in Venezuela, I met a beautiful, dark-skinned girl who fulfilled every dream I had ever had of what a woman should be like. When we made love, I realized for the first time how truly glorious a sexual experience can be. I also felt immense relief to learn that sex was, indeed, just as good as all my shipmates said it was. In fact, sex with the right person was better than anything I'd ever believed possible. In the months and years to come, there would be many other girls in many other ports, but that first love affair left an indelible mark.

Miracle at Muscle Beach

There were other changes in me, too. My interest in bodybuilding and nutrition had steadily grown. Early in my seagoing career, I had acquired a set of weights, and I worked out with them almost every day. I also took regular vitamin supplements at a time when most of my friends would have laughed at the idea if they had known.

By 1949, when I was 16, bodybuilding was still in its infancy, but it had become the focal point of my life. I felt compelled to go to Santa Monica, California, and an area known as "Muscle Beach," which was the indisputable capital of bodybuilding in the U.S. and a mecca for bodybuilders all over North America.

I went ashore with $600, which was a sizable chunk of money at the time. I moved into a rooming house where eight other bodybuilders were living and where room and board cost $10 a week. For almost six months, I did nothing but train on the beach and work out in an old gym known as "The Dungeon." I became close friends with people like Vic Tanny, the owner of the gym; his brother, Armand, who won the "Mr. U.S.A." and "Mr. America" titles in 1950; George Eiferman, "Mr. America" of 1949; and Joe Gold, founder of Gold's Gym and World Gym.

I learned a lot from all of them, but it was Armand Tanny who first taught me to wrestle and laid the groundwork for a fabulous, undreamed-of new career.

"Ray soaked up everything I taught him like a sponge, and he improved upon it," Armand was kind enough to say of me later. "Ray's undying will, fierce determination and discipline to be the best made him a world champion wrestler in only a few short years."

At the time, though, what I really wanted was just to stay at Muscle Beach. When my $600 was gone, I lived on $25 a week in unemployment benefits as long as I could. And even when that was exhausted, I couldn't bring myself to leave. I swiped cans of tuna from local grocery stores to keep from starving while I stretched my stay to a few more weeks.

Finally, I told Armand and Joe Gold that I had no choice. I had to go back to sea to earn a living. But they said, "No, you don't. With some coaching, you can become a professional wrestler."

Me, a wrestler? I couldn't believe it at first. But they had both been pro wrestlers themselves and they saw potential in me that ordinary people couldn't have seen.

From that point on, my whole life changed with whirlwind suddenness. A miraculous transformation was starting to take place.

Facing the "Mean and Ugly"

After several months of rigorous wrestling training by Joe and Armand and a few small-time bouts in California, I went back to New York to try to get my wrestling career off the ground. It was early 1950 and I had just turned 17 years old.

At the time, television was taking the country by storm, but it offered nothing remotely resembling the variety of TV today. In New York, the nation's largest media market, television consisted mostly of Milton Berle and professional wrestling. Televised wrestling matches meant big money for the participants, but the cards were controlled by three brothers named Rudy, Ernie and Amil Dusek. The Dusek brothers were not only promoters; all three had also been professional wrestlers, and they had one helluva reputation.

I'd heard them described as the "meanest, ugliest, toughest" human beings in the world, and the description was perfectly accurate except for one thing. I'm still not totally convinced they were human.

The first time I walked into the Dusek brothers' office, Ernie bellowed out at me in a voice like a foghorn: "Whadda you want, kid?"

"I want to wrestle," I managed to bellow back at him.

"We're busy," snarled another Dusek brother. "Come back tomorrow."

So I did. When I came back the next day, they were sitting around in a cloud of smoke, puffing big, stinking stogies, and they looked just as nasty as ever.

"You think you're pretty strong, huh, kid?" Ernie asked sarcastically.

As a matter of fact, I did. I'd celebrated my birthday by doing 30 reps with 300 pounds on the squat in Vic Tanny's Dungeon. So I immediately snapped, "Yes, sir!"

"We'll see," Ernie growled. "You hold your arm out here and I'm going to try to pull it down with two fingers. I want to see how well you can resist."

This is going to be a piece of cake, I thought to myself. As he pushed down on my arm, I pushed up with everything I had. All at once, Ernie let my arm go and I hit myself in the face so hard I blacked my eye. They all laughed uproariously, and I learned another valuable lesson.

I had a shiner for a week, but I also had a job wrestling professionally on TV.

Mom's Priceless Advice

One of the bonuses of being back in New York was being reunited with my family. After watching me wrestle on TV three times a week – mostly getting my brains beat out at first – my mother sat me down and gave me a short lecture. For a long time, I didn't fully understand what she was trying to tell me, but now I know it may have been the most valuable piece of financial advice I ever received.

"Ray," she said, "look at you. You're a big star on television, but you're being taken advantage of. You're getting injured and you don't have anything to show for it."

"But Mom," I said, "I'm making good money."

"Don't tell me how much you make, Ray," she said. "Tell me how much you save."

I don't know how many millions of dollars I ran through before the full wisdom of that remark finally sank in on me. Over a period of nearly 20 years, I wrestled close to 5,000 professional bouts. I was world heavyweight wrestling champion from 1956 to 1959 and shared the world tag-team title in 1956. I made and spent more money during that period than lots of people see in a lifetime, and after that, I enjoyed financial success again and again in various fields. But I wouldn't have anything to show for all this today if I hadn't learned to follow my mother's advice.

New Profession, New Name

Ever since I first left home at 13, I'd been caught up in a kind of ongoing identity crisis, and as I moved into professional wrestling, I also added a new chapter to that continuing story. During three years as a merchant seaman, I had lived and worked under the name Paul Davis, but Walter Bookbinder was the name I'd been born with, and my promoter quickly let me know that it wasn't a suitable name for a pro wrestler.

"You've got to change it to something short and snappy – something people can remember easily," he said.

After giving it a lot of thought, I decided to adopt my grandfather's surname, which was also my mother's maiden name – Stern. I loved my grandfather deeply and thought of it as a tribute to him. Since the promoters wanted a one-syllable first name to go with it, I chose Ray. Ray Stern. I liked the sound of that.

My career as a professional wrestler blossomed quickly,

primarily because I had some great mentors. One person, in particular, who helped me immeasurably was "Nature Boy" Buddy Rogers, one of the most innovative showmen in the history of the sport. If you wanted to see ability, a great body and tremendous athleticism, Buddy was your man. He had it all, and thanks to him and the work he did with me, I was transformed into a top pro in the space of a single year.

I was highly motivated to succeed, so I also trained hard on my own, keeping my body weight at a lean but muscular 210 pounds. I also got plenty of rest and made sure I had lots of protein in my diet. Since I didn't make much money at first, I couldn't afford to buy a lot of expensive meat, but I managed to strike a deal with a butcher's school to buy the cuts of meat they practiced on at a very low price, and that solved the problem.

As I gained exposure on TV, I quickly became known throughout the wrestling world for my aerial, acrobatic style, which featured a lot of drop kicks and flying head scissors. Because of this unusual style, some people started calling me by the nickname "Thunder." The promoters and TV announcers picked up on it, and soon the "name game" got carried a step further. I became Ray "Thunder" Stern, and the name has stuck with me ever since.

Looking for Something More

In 1954, I returned to Los Angeles as one of the nation's top wrestling stars, appearing on television in the LA area three nights a week. It was hard to believe how far I had come in such a short time. I had gained polish, wisdom, experience, recognition and financial success. I was on the way to the very pinnacle of my profession, and every day brought me to new plateaus.

By 1956, I had won the two top titles in U.S. heavyweight wrestling. I had also won the adulation of wrestling fans from coast to coast. I had made – and continued to make – a lot of money. And yet, I had this unshakeable feeling deep inside that life had a great deal more in store for me. Although I'd been making my own way for more than 10 years, I was still a very young guy, but I already realized that I couldn't keep wrestling forever.

That same flamboyant, aerobatic style that made me so popular with the public was taking a terrific toll on my body. If I hadn't been in such superb physical shape, the toll would have been even greater. I knew that sooner or later I needed to establish myself in some kind of business outside the wrestling ring.

Meanwhile, at age 19, just as I was working my way into the upper echelons of wrestling, I had gotten married to a girl who seemed the fulfillment of all my fondest dreams. She was not only beautiful, but also wholesome, well-educated, cultured and refined – qualities that I longed to associate myself with.

My goals went beyond money and fame alone. I also wanted to mingle with a higher caliber of individuals. I wanted to fit in and be comfortable with people who lived up to those images I had seen in the movies when I was a boy. People who spoke correctly, displayed perfect manners and exuded the kind of class I had always wanted for myself. My first wife exemplified exactly that type of person.

Unfortunately, I discovered too late that I wasn't yet mature enough for a permanent relationship and the commitment it required. I found it impossible to give up the partying and womanizing that had become an ingrained part of my lifestyle. After a year and a half, the marriage ended in separation and divorce.

Launching a New Life

Not long after my first marital breakup, I went to San Francisco to wrestle. One day, at Aquatic Park, I met the most incredibly built woman I'd ever seen. Her name was Clare Hasse, and she was not only gorgeous; she also had a brilliant mind. I could tell she was smarter than I was, but I didn't care. I couldn't get enough of her, and she seemed to like me, too.

But after we'd been hanging out together for several weeks, she stunned me one day by telling me she thought it best if we stopped seeing each other.

"I need to be with someone who's business-minded and going somewhere with his life," she told me calmly. "That means someone with a much more stable career than a professional wrestler."

"But Clare," I protested, "I'm going to be a great success – a real businessman. Just wait and see."

She smiled. "I believe you've got the talent and ability," she said, "and maybe you'll make it someday. But I think it's best for me to find someone who's already there."

We didn't see each other again for months. During that interval, I missed Clare deeply, and as it turned out, she missed me, too. Eventually, we were drawn back together, and by now I think both of us realized how personally right we were for each other. But this time, I also managed to convince her that I was serious about succeeding in business. We were married in 1956 when I was still only 23, and about a year later, we opened our first business together. It was a 2,000-square-foot health club just for women, and it was an instant success. We immediately made plans to expand.

Then, in 1957, we took a huge gamble. We opened the first coed health club in the United States in San Mateo, California. It was such a tremendous overnight success that we soon converted our female-only club in San Francisco to a coed operation, and it, too, took off like a rocket.

On the Crest of a Wave

The coed health club concept took the West Coast by storm, and before long, we were making unbelievable amounts of money. I thought I had earned big bucks as a wrestler, but it had been peanuts compared to this. From one 8,700-square-foot club in San Francisco we took in an average of more than $100,000 a month during 1958-59.

Now that's still a hefty sum of money today, but in the late 1950s, a dollar was worth maybe ten times what it is in the mid-'90s. To give you a frame of reference, the highest-paid stars of major league baseball made around $120,000 a year in those days. And when film star Janet Leigh starred in the classic Alfred Hitchcock thriller, Psycho, which came out about that same time, she was paid $25,000 for her role. Clare and I were making four times that much every month.

We constantly added innovations to keep our facilities at the forefront of the health club craze. We opened the first health club nurseries, which allowed husbands and wives to work out together while their children had supervision and a place to play. We also offered the nation's first exercise classes at our clubs. That was long before the term "aerobics" was ever heard, but the classes featured the same type of cardiovascular-fitness exercises that the Cooper Clinic would popularize a decade later.

When the really big money began to roll in, however, I got a very unpleasant surprise in the form of an extremely big tax bill.

I didn't mind paying my fair share of taxes, but people in the higher income brackets were hit extremely hard in those days. More than ever before, I realized the truth of my mother's admonition to me: "It's not what you make; it's what you save."

I had learned to make lots of money, but now I also had to learn to hang onto it and invest it wisely. I read every book and magazine article I could find relating to taxes and finances. I talked to accountants, other businessmen and anyone else who could help me understand tax laws and how they affected Clare and me.

My conclusion: The time had come to start branching out financially.

Getting Into Real Estate

I had a friend and training partner named Andy Oddstad, whose company, Oddstad Homes, was the nation's 10th largest homebuilder. Through our association, I had learned quite a bit about real estate construction and development, including the fact that real estate investments enjoyed a very favorable tax status at the time, because the properties could be depreciated to offset the income they produced. Now I decided to put some of that information to practical use.

In a fast-growing economy like that on the West Coast, rental property seemed to be an especially promising investment. My first venture into this new field was relatively small – a 12-unit apartment building. But when the building filled with tenants almost immediately, something larger seemed in order.

The next project was three times the size of the first – 36 units – and it, too, was quickly filled to capacity. The cash flow created by these rental properties was little short of fantastic, so I decided to aim still higher. My next building contained 72 units, and all of them were quickly leased.

One of my goals in these ventures was full control of the properties I built. I considered myself a developer, not a passive investor. I drew the rough plans myself to show how I wanted each building to look. Then I subcontracted all the construction work, and when the building was finished, I took over the responsibilities of managing it. This allowed me to control every phase of the project.

From this point on, real estate development became a major part of my life.

A Political Bombshell

With five health clubs in operation, a string of profitable apartment buildings and a new finance company organized to finance our health club memberships, I now had almost 500 people on my various payrolls. I thought I was sitting on top of the world, but what I was actually sitting on was a ticking political timebomb that was just about to explode.

I was about to suffer my first serious financial setback, but it had nothing whatsoever to do with business. It was the result of a vicious political witchhunt. I first learned about it one Sunday morning when I opened the newspaper and saw my name in bold, black headlines, along with the accusation that our clubs were engaged in fraudulent practices and the threat that we would soon be shut down.

The charges against us, of course, were entirely false. At the root of the uproar was California Assemblyman Leo Ryan, who was trying to gain support for a bill he had introduced into the state legislature to prohibit health clubs from selling long-term memberships. The bill would have allowed only month-to-month memberships to be sold, but without being able to sign up members for periods of one, two or three years, the health club industry couldn't have provided the kind of service the public demanded, and the result would've been disastrous.

We made up our minds to fight the bill and hired an aggressive young former lobbyist as our attorney. I also launched a public relations blitz to try to counteract all the vicious, false and damaging stories that were circulating about our clubs. I was determined that nobody was going to wreck my business, but I also realized I was in the fight of my life. I had thought wrestling was tough, but I soon found politics to be tougher. It was like wrestling a pit full of alligators.

After the bill was defeated, Ryan then tried to attack me through the state attorney general's office and by using the press to spread his trumped-up allegations. We almost went bankrupt before we were able to turn the situation around and bring our clubs back to prosperity with such innovative marketing strategies as offering free two-week trial memberships and programs designed to help patrons lose up to 15 pounds during that two-week period.

Leo Ryan, incidentally, went on to become a U.S. congressman from California. But his career and his life ended tragically when his insatiable drive for publicity took him to Jonestown, Guyana, to confront the Reverend Jim Jones and his cult followers. He died there, along with hundreds of others.

Learning and Planning

After the dispute was finally settled and my business was saved, I looked back on the painful struggle I had just gone through and tried to draw something positive from it. Again, I had learned some important lessons, not only about business and politics, but about life, too.

I learned, for example, that success can breed cockiness and overconfidence, and that no matter how successful you become, the danger of failure is always there. I learned to beware of people who feed your ego by telling you how brilliant you are. Compliments can inspire you to greater heights, but they can also delude you into becoming lazy and complacent. The ego can be a powerful ally or a deadly enemy, depending on how you use it.

The process of succeeding in life is partly based on accumulating knowledge, wisdom and experience. But it's also based in part on minimizing the number of stupid mistakes you make. Even the shrewdest, smartest people can screw up when they behave impulsively, foolishly or imprudently.

My emerging business philosophy was to build for the long term, rather than to follow the tempting route of fast-buck tactics and get-rich-quick schemes. For instance, after the health clubs were solidly back on their feet, I leased out the facilities to a company called European Spas. The new company took over the day-to-day operation of the facilities, while I was freed to pursue new opportunites. But I retained ownership of the clubs in addition to gaining long-term income potential.

It was at this point in my life that I began to discover how important advance planning can be. I started training myself to think and plan in terms of 5- or 10-year increments. Just as a superior physique can't be built overnight, neither can a successful business venture. Having a great body, like achieving great wealth and success, comes only through discipline, commitment to your goals, and the ability to plan decisively and think positively.

I've continued to prepare for the future through multi-year planning ever since. Planning not only allows you to chart a practical course toward a specific goal; it also helps you avoid mistakes and blunders along the way. All plans are subject to modification, of course, but they give you a blueprint from which to work.

Soaring to New Heights

Ever since my first plane ride at age 19, I've been in love with flying. That first flight took place in Florida in a J-3 Piper Cub owned by fellow wrestler Billy Darnell, and the instant we were airborne, I felt a tremendous surge of excitement. From that moment on, I knew I wanted to be a pilot.

A short time later, after just two weeks of flying lessons, I got my pilot's license. Of course, airplanes weren't nearly as sophisticated or complicated in the early '50s as they are today, and the licensing requirements weren't nearly as stringent. I had mastered a few fundamentals, but I didn't realize how little I really knew about flying until I almost killed myself a few times. One emergency landing I made with the help of car headlights on an abandoned airstrip near Bonham, Texas, was especially thrilling.

With practice, however, I became an excellent pilot. And, typically for me in those wild and woolly early days, I developed a major interest in aerobatics. After all, it tied right in with the unique wrestling style that had earned me the nickname "Thunder."

After Clare and I moved to Dallas, I worked long and hard to perfect my aerobatic skills. I bought two aerobatic planes in Czechoslovakia and even brought the Czech aerobatics champion to Dallas to train me. I placed as high as fourth in the unlimited division of the national competitions and was twice chosen as an alternate on the U.S. Aerobatic Team for worldwide competition.

I once got in trouble with the FAA and had my licenses revoked as a result of a false report that I was practicing aerobatics outside my designated practice area. Not only did I have to wait a year before I could re-apply, but I also would have to take and pass all the tests all over again. Although I had logged more than 6,000 hours of flying time, I was so disgusted that I made up my mind to quit. But then a friend told me something that caused me to rethink my decision.

"Most businessmen would give anything for the flying experience you have," he said. "And you're going to give all that up?

Don't be ridiculous!"

As it turned out, I repassed the tests and re-qualified as everything from a student pilot on up to an airline transport pilot within a single month. It's a good thing I did. Otherwise, I would've missed out on a phenomenal new financial opportunity.

You see, as so often happens when I become intensely interested in something, flying was destined to become far more than a mere hobby or avocation for me. It was also to lead to another major business incentive and the eventual formation of another multi-million-dollar commercial enterprise – SternAir, Inc.

From One Jet to a Fleet

For years, one of my big dreams had been to own a Lear jet. This magnificent plane is the "Rolls Royce of private aircraft." It possesses speed and altitude capabilities, custom features, superior design and quality workmanship that make it synonymous with prestige and performance. But the price tag of a Lear was in the millions, and I wasn't flying enough in my existing businesses to justify the tremendous expense.

Not long after the unpleasantness with the FAA, however, a fantastic idea occurred to me. If I set up my own company and kept the Lear busy with charter, cargo and/or air ambulance services when I wasn't using it for something else, I could both justify the expense and possibly end up making significant money on the deal as well.

When SternAir started operations in the mid-'70s, word spread quickly about the unusual service we offered – we would fly anything or anybody anywhere and under any circumstances – and the business grew faster than I ever thought possible. Before long, the SternAir fleet included five Lears and two Falcon jets.

With this many planes, I quickly discovered that it cost a bundle to keep these expensive jets in tip-top condition. In considering how to cut service costs, I came up with another dynamite idea: I would hire a staff of expert mechanics and open my own service center where I could not only service my own aircraft but other people's, too.

When obstacles developed – and I had learned by now that they always do – I looked for innovative ways to get around them. Usually, I found them. One of the best examples of this was when I ran head-on into the unfair and monopolistic system under which the French company that manufactured landing gear parts for the Falcon jets refused to sell those parts to anyone but Falcon Jet Corporation itself.

I decided to take the kind of typically direct action that's always worked best for me. I flew to France and met for several hours with the chairman of the landing gear company. I told him, as politely and diplomatically as I could, that what he was doing was considered an unfair restraint of trade and could cause him problems with the U.S. government.

Within weeks, his company was supplying me with all the parts I needed and I was overhauling dozens of Falcon landing gears at a cost of $150,000 per set of three. This meant millions of dollars worth of business to SternAir, and the demand for landing gear service grew so fast that I had to hire many additional technicians, engineers and pilots.

Another prime example of curbing monopolistic practices to cut expenses and raise profits came when I changed my fuel-buying practices. At many airports, one company supplies all the jet fuel and basically charges whatever it wants to charge. But I decided the price was too high at the airport where SternAir was located, so I negotiated a new deal with an outside supplier who agreed to sell me all the fuel I needed at one-third the other supplier's price. Since a Lear or Falcon consumes 250 to 350 gallons of jet fuel an hour, the savings have been astronomical.

Big Doings in "Big D"

I've already mentioned that I moved my base of operations from the West Coast to Dallas in the early 1970s. The catalyst for the move came when the Federal Housing Adminstration began offering various real estate properties for sale to the highest bidder. The sale prices were usually well below market value, which could mean a tidy profit if an investor was fortunate enough to land one. And I was.

The property I acquired from the FHA was the Wedgewood Towers, a magnificent 300-unit, high-rise apartment building on eight acres of land in Dallas. I had already been in the real estate business, but now I was in it in a bigger way than ever before.

At first, I thought I would commute from San Francisco to Dallas once or twice a month to keep tabs on my investment.

But I found myself increasingly attracted to this fast-growing Texas city, and so did Clare. For one thing, nearby Fort Worth was a mecca for aerobatic flying. But the main thing was that the Dallas area was alive with incredible opportunities. In many ways, the atmosphere was much like it had been in California just after World War II. For someone with nerve, an entrepreneurial spirit and money to invest, "Big D" represented a golden opportunity. And I believed I fit that description to a tee.

So I made a momentous decision: I'd move to Dallas and build a penthouse atop the Wedgewood Towers as a home. For the time being, I'd also keep my home in San Francisco and fly there every few weeks to take care of business. I made up my mind to go where the action was, and I've never regretted it. There's a wonderful, exuberant, sky's-the-limit feeling about Dallas that's hard to match anywhere else.

In this atmosphere, Clare and I formulated plans for the health club of our dreams. It was this club that would help make exercise and fitness household words across America – and make us millions more dollars in the process.

We intended to incorporate two unique features into our new state-of-the-art fitness center. First, it would feature the first racquetball facilities in the Dallas area. Second, it would include the first coed gym anywhere outside California. People said that idea would never sell in "Baptist country" like Texas. No conservative Texas husband was going to want his wife working out in a gym filled with other guys, they warned.

We went ahead with the project anyway. Based on our California experience, we were convinced that Dallas was ready for this type of club, and we were right. Our dream club had six racquetball courts that were constantly in use. They had glass back walls, and a restaurant and bar were located between the courts, so that patrons could watch the players while they were eating and drinking. The idea was a smash hit, and our club became one of the best-known "in" spots in the city.

An Expensive Mistake

I firmly believe that honesty is the best policy, both in your business dealings and in your personal relationships. That's why I've never tried to hide my mistakes, only to benefit from them. And along with my considerable business successes have come a few mistakes that were real doozies.

A few years after scoring big with our super fitness center in Dallas, I started feeling burned-out and bored, as I have periodically all my life. I knew the best cure for this condition was a new challenge, preferably one involving financial promise as well as excitement. I found it in the commodities and currency markets, where almost incalculable amounts of money were being made in the late 1970s.

My routine as a commodities speculator went like this: My broker would call each morning about 8:45 a.m., just as my cook was bringing my breakfast into the bedroom. For the next hour or two, I would buy and sell just about anything you can imagine – Mexican pesos, livestock and agricultural futures, German marks, Swiss francs, etc.

It was utterly incredible how fast the money rolled in. But it was even more incredible how easy it was. I had spent a lot of my life working 16 hours a day, and now I couldn't help but wonder why. My profits were running as high as $45,000 a day, and I was hardly having to lift a finger!

Then the unthinkable happened. Almost overnight, the bottom fell out of the commodities and currency markets, and I lost virtually everything I'd made. I'd let myself get so caught up in the euphoria of what I was doing that I'd forgotten how suddenly everything can go sour.

It was probably the costliest financial mistake of my life. But once more, I vowed it would be a lesson I'd never forget. To hang onto a fortune in today's volatile economic conditions, you have to guard it carefully and invest it wisely. In my own case, I made the decision to never again become heavily involved in an investment over which I had no control. From this point on, I would risk my money only in investments that could be thoroughly researched in advance, then monitored from start to finish.

I bounced back from the commodities market mess by building the magnificent Claremont, a high-rise development encompassing 360 condominium units, offices, a health spa and gym, indoor and outdoor swimming pools, steam rooms, saunas and jogging track. I topped it off with a 15,000-square-foot penthouse for Clare and me.

Training "Miss Universe"

Even with all the business successes I've enjoyed, my enthusiasm for bodybuilding and physical fitness has never wavered.

One of my most satisfying accomplishments came in November 1993 when my training program helped Monica Rios win the AAU title of "Miss Universe" – the greatest honor a female bodybuilder can attain.

Monica was an attractive woman of 35 when I first began working with her. But she was considerably overweight and out of condition. She ate the same high-fat foods that most Americans eat and knew very little about nutrition. She was also a three-pack-a-day cigarette smoker and consumed alcohol on a regular basis.

Her main interest when we first met was in improving her nutrition in order to lose 30 or 35 pounds, and she accomplished this in a fairly short period of time. This initial success made Monica want to do more to improve herself, and one thing led to another. She started a comprehensive exercise program. She quit smoking. She stopped drinking. And after a while, people around the gym started saying, "You look so good you ought to go into competitive bodybuilding."

Monica had shown by now that she had the willpower and dedication it takes to do extraordinary things. I agreed to serve as her trainer, and a short time later, she entered the AAU "Miss Texas" contest and placed second. A few months later, she placed third in the "Miss U.S.A" competition. This might have been enough to satisfy most people, but Monica kept right on working until she won the "Miss Universe" title in Atlantic City.

Today, at 41, Monica is the personification of beauty, health and vitality. Her body is the envy of most 20-year-olds, and the amazing thing is that she's still getting better. I believe she can continue to improve herself physically for at least another 20 or 25 years. In the meantime, she is also living proof of what an "ordinary" person can do to turn his or her life completely around.

It was when my friends and associates saw what Monica had accomplished under my training and supervision that they began to say to me: "Ray, you ought to write a book about your approach to total health and fitness, so that thousands of other people can benefit from Monica's example."

But although bodybuilding has always remained my "first love," and its benefits have carried me through every type of crisis imaginable, I didn't want to do a book strictly about bodybuilding or exercise. I wanted a book that would present the complete "big picture" on how to achieve better health, greater fitness, more success and satisfaction and longer life. My decades of working out have helped me to look, feel and perform my best and have also made it possible for me to bounce back from defeat and disappointment again and again, to turn misfortune into fortune. But excellent nutrition, a long-standing awareness of the importance of maintaining health and preventing disease, plus the will to resist damaging lifestyle habits have also been major assets in my successes.

Another thing that's allowed me to accomplish so many things in so many different fields of endeavor is a positive attitude and an inquiring nature. When I was a kid, I did things that other kids only fantasize about doing. At an age when most young guys are content to spend their time and energy drinking, carousing and chasing girls, I was building a fortune and becoming a multi-millionaire. When I reached my middle years, the time when most people think they should start slowing down, I was looking for new worlds to conquer. As the Bible says, "Seek and ye shall find."

Act Your Age? But Why?

And now that I'm in my 60s, I intend to continue that trend. I refuse to say, "I'm too old to do that." I'm not going to stop doing anything I want to do or taking any risk I want to take simply because I'm not 25 or 30 or 40 years old anymore. I'm thoroughly convinced that I'm actually younger in a biological sense than lots of people half my chronological age.

I want you to feel that way, too. Section by section, chapter by chapter, that feeling is what this book is all about. For close to 50 years, I've been a sort of "walking research project" in areas ranging from business and high finance to nutrition, exercise and physical fitness. This book gives you an opportunity to take advantage of all I've learned and proved by trial and error in my personal research.

I've discovered that you can create your own luck – at any age. I've found you can affect your environment, rather than being trapped and overwhelmed by it. I've learned the wisdom of always keeping your options open; if you do, there's no mistake you can't overcome. I know first-hand the benefits of dealing with people and situations with honesty, forthrightness and creativity. I've proved the principles of working, saving, building, planning, dreaming and taking care of yourself. These are the ingredients of which wealth and long life are made.

I've been a gambler and a risk-taker all my life. Yet I've never bought a single lottery ticket and never will. Playing the lottery isn't risk-taking. It's only self-defeating self-delusion. Put that buck you're tempted to spend on the lottery into the bank instead. Better yet, invest it in something sensible and controllable. Be patient and wait for it to multiply.

You've got time. So you're over 50 – so what? You've got plenty of time to do what's important. The trick is to start doing it. There's no way you should take on a 30-year mortgage at this stage of the game, but there was no way you should've done that when you were 25. Thirty-year mortgages at any age are bad investments that can cost hundreds of thousands of dollars in unnecessary interest. Go for 10 or 15 years instead. With the money you save, you can buy a Cadillac and a condo and travel around the world a few times.

Retirement? Sure, I may retire some day. Matter of fact, I've been "retiring" periodically for years – discarding one type of endeavor for something I find more appealing or financially attractive at that particular point. This is the only kind of "retirement" I'm interested in.

I'm a fortunate guy, but I wasn't born fortunate. Nobody is, really. Good fortune – like good health and long life – comes to those who have the willpower to reach for it and the resolve to hang on once they've grasped it.

It can be yours. It's high time you realized that.

"Your nutrition can determine how you look, act and feel; whether you are grouchy or cheerful, homely or beautiful, physiologically and even psychologically young or old; whether you think clearly or are confused, enjoy your work or make it a drudgery, increase your earning power or stay in an economic rut."
—ADELLE DAVIS

CHAPTER 4

Diet and Nutrition for Health, Long Life and Appearance

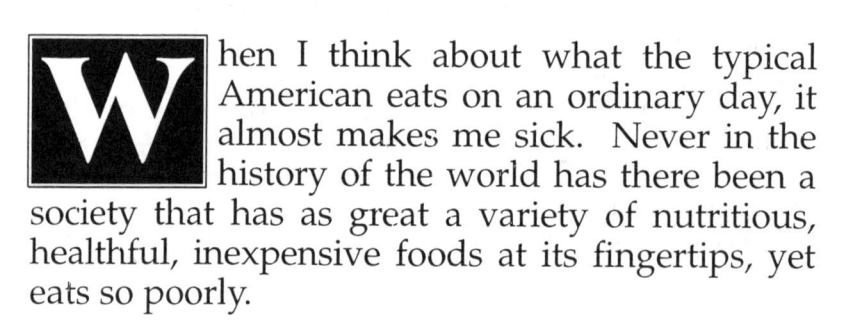

When I think about what the typical American eats on an ordinary day, it almost makes me sick. Never in the history of the world has there been a society that has as great a variety of nutritious, healthful, inexpensive foods at its fingertips, yet eats so poorly.

The rate of drug addiction in our country is shocking, but our national addiction to greasy, salty, sugary "junk food" is a thousand times worse because it affects so many more people. We are literally a nation of "junk food junkies"!

As a result, tens of millions of us are literally eating ourselves to death.

It's utterly tragic that 71 percent of all the men, women and children in this country are obese. When I first read that statistic, I couldn't believe it. I thought, "This has got to be a typographical error." But I was wrong. It's true.

Just think of it. This means that more than seven out of every 10 Americans are overweight. That's close to three-fourths of the citizens of what has to be the most health-conscious country on earth. This means that only 29 percent – barely over one-quarter of our population – maintains a normal or below-normal weight.

"Dietary Suicide"

There's a persistent popular notion that obesity is usually the result of over-nutrition. That is, we simply eat more nourishing food than our bodies can use and we store the excess as fat. Sometimes this is true. But much more often, obese people are also actually suffering from malnutrition. They undoubtedly overeat, but they also eat nutritionally deficient foods. As a result, they leave their fat bodies literally starved for vital nutrients.

Terrible as it is, the worst thing about this situation isn't the people who are being killed off many years – and even decades – before their time by their horrible diet. The worst thing is that there's no logical reason for this to happen. Otherwise intelligent people are committing "dietary suicide" every day, and it just doesn't make sense.

With the advancements we've made in food production and food processing, along with our increased awareness of human nutritional needs and dangers, there's less excuse than ever before for so many millions of people to be getting fat and staying that way.

So why are close to 180,000,000 of us overweight? Why are we dying by the hundreds of thousands each year from coronary heart disease, strokes, diabetes and various types of cancer that can be linked directly to our faulty, fat-laden diet?

There are only two primary reasons, and both are deceptively simple: (1) We eat too much of the wrong kinds of food, and (2) we don't get enough exercise.

Like it or not, that's the way it is. But there's an important underlying factor in this scenario.

Adrift in Confusion

As highly educated as we are as a nation, we're still incredibly ignorant about nutrition. Not stupid, mind you, just ignorant. Uninformed.

Unfortunately, many "experts" are ignorant and uninformed, too. Their ignorance compounds the problem and makes it hard to get reliable information. The media is overflowing with conflicting and/or misleading "facts" about nutrition, based on the latest findings by "experts." Much of this misinformation can be hazardous to your health and mine.

News reports about nutritional research have an infuriating habit of contradicting themselves. One report implies we should be eating more polyunsaturated fat, so people give up butter with the idea that they can use all the "soft" margarine they want. Another article says we should be eating more monounsaturated fat, so they load up on olive oil just to be on the "safe side."What we really need to do is drastically reduce our intake of all kinds of fats, but this message frequently gets lost in the confusion.

A small amount of fat in the diet is vital to good health because of the essential fatty acids it contains. But the average American gets 10 to 20 times the amount of fat he or she needs. And there is virtually no danger of any of us becoming "fat-deficient" – if there is such a thing – since tiny amounts of fat occur naturally in almost all types of vegetable matter and in much higher concentrations in meat, fish and other animal products.

Doctors, meanwhile, as mentioned earlier, haven't kept pace with the explosion in nutritional knowledge. They see their responsibility as treating specific illnesses in their special fields, not as dispensers of information on general nutrition. And as incredible as it seems, many nutritionists – the very professionals who are supposed to be the utmost authority on dietary needs – don't know their asparagus from their elbow macaroni when it comes to designing a diet for optimum health and longevity.

Beware of Obese "Experts"

I attended a lecture by a nutritionist not long ago – a grossly overweight nutritionist, I might add. (You know, I've always believed if somebody's handing out advice on something, he or she should "look the part." For instance, I wouldn't be particularly interested in taking financial advice from a banker with holes in his shoes, or advice about bodybuilding from a 97-pound weakling. And so, to me, the advice of an obese nutritionist is immediately suspect.)

Anyway, this particular "expert," who had years of experience and a master's degree in nutrition, recommended a basic diet of 1,500 calories a day for an active woman of medium build, which is about right. But then I asked her how those calories should be broken down – how many from fat, how many from carbohydrates, how many from protein? – and she said it didn't matter.

"Fifteen hundred calories is 1,500 calories," she said.

"Are you trying to tell me that 1,500 calories from egg whites and baked fish has the same effect on the body as 1,500 calories from candy bars?" I asked.

"That's right," she said. "A calorie is a calorie. It makes no difference where it comes from."

I could only shake my head in disbelief. It's precisely this kind of thinking – or, more accurately, lack of thinking – that produces so many malnourished fat people.

The Amazing Supermarket

If a layman with no nutritional training made a statement like this, it could be charged off to ignorance. We could just assume the person didn't know any better. But when a professional nutritionist spouts this kind of nonsense, it can only be defined as pompous stupidity.

Try living on candy bars for a while, and you'll know what I mean.

If you intend to make the most of your second 50 years – or even have a second 50 – it's time to stop listening to such hogwash. The time to end your ignorance and your dependence on "experts" who don't know what they're talking about is right now!

One of the first things you need to become aware of is what amazing foods are out there in the marketplace today. And I'm not talking about the exotic products in expensive health food stores, either. Everything you need for complete nutritional health is right there in your neighborhood supermarket.

Within the past five or six years, a tremendous revolution has taken place in the American food industry. From the farmers who grow the crops and raise the livestock to the processors and packagers of the finished consumer products, the emphasis is on healthy, low-fat foods.

Walk into the typical supermarket today and you'll find literally hundreds of new products that weren't there a few years ago: sugar-free and fat-free desserts, non-fat butter substitutes, fat-free mayonnaise and salad dressings, fat-free sour cream, non-caloric sweeteners, salt substitutes, cheese with 50 percent less fat or no fat at all, meats and fish with 98, 99, even 100 percent of the measurable fat removed.

Getting the Fat Out

Only a few years ago, commercial bakers seemed to load all their products with fat. Breads, cakes, cookies and pastries contained high percentages of shortening, lard, beef tallow and tropical oils. But now low-fat or no-fat whole-grain breads and cereals are the rule, not the exception. Non-fat and reduced fat cookies are also commonplace – some of them deceptively rich-tasting. If you absolutely have to snack, baked tortilla chips and potato chips are also available, in both salted and unsalted versions.

And over in the produce section is an ever-expanding array of fresh fruits and vegetables that would do justice to the tables of royalty. Virtually all of them are bursting with energizing carbohydrates and health-building vitamins and minerals, yet contain practically no fat and a minimum of calories. Of all the foods in that produce section, the only one I'd strongly suggest avoiding is avocadoes, which I regard as one of "nature's mistakes." An avocado contains more fat and calories than any other vegetable or fruit – almost as much, ounce for ounce, as regular sour cream.

The problem is no longer that healthful foods aren't available in abundance. It's not that following a healthful, low-fat diet involves great pain or sacrifice. It's just that most Americans are either unaware of all of today's many options or they choose to ignore them.

Greasy Kid (and Adult) Stuff

The purveyors of "junk food" spend billions of dollars each year advertising their products on TV, but how long has it been since you saw a TV ad promoting fresh fruits and vegetables or natural grains or lean meat and fish? The companies that spend the big bucks are those selling greasy snacks, fast foods, sugar-laden cereals, candy and other sweets. Many of their messages are aimed at teenagers and kids. Is it any wonder that our younger generation has such appalling eating habits? Or that so many kids are overweight and out of shape?

Look at what they consume:

French fries. Pizza. Nachos. Fried chicken. Fried fish. Hamburgers. Hotdogs. Chips and dips. Tacos. Hot wings. Fried cheese. Peanuts and peanut butter. Buttered (and often cocoanut-oiled) popcorn. Ice cream. Doughnuts. Pastries. Chocolate bars. Sugary soft drinks.

If you want a graphic example of what kids shouldn't eat, check out what they're serving at the nearest school cafeteria. Instead of taking the opportunity to see that children get at least one nutritious, well-balanced, healthful meal each schoolday, most cafeterias do their very best to imitate the fast-food chains. The result: too many calories, too much salt, too much sugar and far too much fat. Except for the catsup on fries, the lettuce and pickles on hamburgers, the tomato sauce on pizza and spaghetti, and the filling in pies, fruits and vegetables are almost non-existent.

And in our hurried, harried world, adults rarely set a good example. As a rule, parents are just as nutritionally bankrupt as their kids. Dad's idea of a good breakfast is an "Egg McMuffin" and coffee. Mom's version of a healthy lunch is a trip to an all-you-can-eat salad bar, heavy on the cheese, bacon bits, pasta and creamy ranch dressing. Supper is a bucket of "extra crispy" from KFC or a Pizza Hut "Bigfoot" in a greasy box. Dinner at a "nice" restaurant is a big slab of lasagna or some fettucini Alfredo (which I've heard described as "a heart attack on a plate"), or fajitas dripping in oil and served with guacamole, or a juicy steak and a baked potato swimming in butter and sour cream. Add a few beers, a few glasses of wine, a couple of margaritas or piña coladas, top it off with cheesecake or double-chocolate cake for dessert and you've got an adults-only version of our national nutritional disaster.

What it all boils down to (and it might be better for you if you did boil it for a while to get some of the grease out) is huge amounts of fat, sugar, salt and empty calories.

It's Easier Than You Think

Most of this stuff tastes good. I have to admit it. But it's poison to your body. Taken in large daily doses, foods like these are a ticket to obesity, clogged arteries, broken health, early disease, premature disability – and death. Making them the mainstays of your diet is simply incompatible with good health and long life.

There's no way around this fact: Sound nutrition has to be one of the major cornerstones of your daily routine if you expect to have a healthy, happy, productive second 50 years. This doesn't mean you can never have another "Big Mac" or another piece of Colonel Sanders' chicken. It doesn't mean you can't occasionally indulge in a slice of pizza or an order of fries. What it does mean is that, if you're a bona fide "junk food junkie," you have to change your basic eating patterns. You have to adopt a nutritional lifestyle that builds health instead of tearing it down.

And my goal in this chapter is to prove to you that this is simpler, easier and less expensive than you think.

For one thing, you can forget about costly diet pills and "magic" weight-loss formulas. You can forget about starving yourself or following kook diets where you eat nothing but grapefruit and boiled eggs or where you have to cut out all carbohydrates. You can also forget about being enslaved by a nutritional regimen that's punitive or highly restrictive. In my opinion, all these approaches are self-defeating and doomed to failure.

Food doesn't have to be unhealthy in order to taste good. Enjoying good food is one of the true pleasures of life. There's no need to give up that pleasure. All you have to do is refocus it a little.

Fat – Public Enemy No. 1

The number-one dietary villain in America is fat. If the truth were known, I suspect fat kills and disables far more people in an average year than even cigarette smoking. It's a silent killer. It gives little or no warning until the damage is done. We put cautionary labels on tobacco products, but not on frankfurters, pork chops, margarine or cheese. Most Americans are confused about fat. Millions of its potential victims don't have a clue about what kind of harm their high-fat diet is doing to them. The vast majority of them have no concept of how much fat they really eat.

Most people who eat a lot of fat believe they'd miss it terribly if it were excluded from their food. But fat actually adds no flavor, only calories and cholesterol. It has some bearing on the texture of food, but has absolutely no taste of its own.

There are three major types of fat – saturated, monounsaturated and polyunsaturated. Most medical research indicates that saturated fat is probably the most harmful to human health.

Our main source of saturated fat is animal foods – meat, fowl, fish, eggs, milk, cheese, butter, etc. But some vegetable fats, such as palm and cocoanut oils, are also highly saturated. And even the most highly unsaturated vegetable fats can be converted into saturated fats during processing.

The simplest way to identify a saturated fat, such as lard or beef tallow, is that it stays solid at room temperature and melts only when heated. Monounsaturated fats, such as olive oil, are liquid at room temperature, but turn cloudy and become semi-liquid under refrigeration. Polyunsaturated fats, such as corn oil, safflower oil or canola oil, remain liquid both at room temperature and in the refrigerator.

In the bloodstream, fats – particularly the saturated kind – are converted into cholesterol. The body gets rid of some cholesterol by breaking it down in the liver and excreting it, but when too much fat is eaten, excess cholesterol molecules lodge in artery walls and damage them, creating thick, rough lesions. Over time, these build up and form obstructions that restrict blood flow in the arteries. When an artery becomes blocked by these restrictions, blood clots can form and cut off the blood supply to part of the heart or brain. This is what causes heart attacks or strokes.

Cut Fat to a Minimum

After decades of research and many conflicting theories, the debate still rages on over which kinds of fat are most harmful and which ones are potentially beneficial. But almost all health authorities now agree that the typical American diet is far too high in fat, period. Whether it's saturated or unsaturated, the simple fact is, we eat much too much of it.

Many Americans get 45 or 50 percent – or more – of their daily calorie intake from fat. The American Heart Association recommends lowering this amount drastically, to no more than 30 percent of total calories from fat, and no more than 10 percent from saturated fat.

That's definitely a step in the right direction. But in my opinion, it doesn't go far enough. If you and I want to protect ourselves from heart disease – the nation's number–one killer – we need to do more. If we seriously intend to remain active and healthy for a century or more, it's vital to cut our fat intake much further. And instead of wasting time wondering and worrying

kinds of fat are less harmful, my approach is to cut
an absolute minimum.

y fat consumption to no more than 10 percent of my
alories, with 30 percent of my calories coming from
protein and 60 percent from complex carbohydrates. On the
3,000-calorie-per-day diet I follow as a bodybuilder, that means
no more than 300 calories can come from fat. This figures out to
about 33 grams of fat (at nine calories per gram) per day. Lots of
people have eaten twice that much fat by the time they leave the
breakfast table in the morning – usually without even giving it a
second thought.

To illustrate how little fat 33 grams actually is, consider that
a half-cup of heavy cream contains 47 grams of fat. A half-cup
of butter contains 90 grams, or almost three times my daily
"allowable." Just one "Big Mac" with fries would exceed my
entire quota of fat for a whole day.

Yet I never feel hungry or deprived. I actually eat five meals
a day, rather than just three, without exceeding my fat quota. I
have all the energy I need for an active, busy lifestyle, plus two
hours of strenuous exercise a day. And I never gain weight.

Magic, you say? Witchcraft? Hocus-pocus? Not at all. Just
common sense and a little self-discipline.

You can do it, too. I'm going to tell you how.

Protein Without Fat

Pursuing an active, aggressive lifestyle at any age requires
large amounts of protein. When you're past 50, your need for
protein becomes even greater. Protein not only provides long-
term, slow-burning energy, but is also essential for healing
injuries and maintaining healthy muscle tissue. It's the stuff
your skin, internal organs, brain, hair and even fingernails are
made of. Every cell depends on it to function normally and
repair itself. But muscles contain more protein than any other
part of the body.

Without an adequate supply of protein, the body quickly
begins to lose lean muscle mass. If you want to see the results of
a radical low-protein diet, just look at pictures of the survivors
of Hitler's concentration camps. There were definitely no problems with overweight there.

You also grow old on the days you don't have enough protein. Since your body structure is largely made up of protein, an

inadequate supply can cause you to age with distressing speed. If you're protein-deficient, you're aging prematurely. You can bet on it. You can also bet that you feel hungry a good part of the time because of low blood sugar.

And unlike fat, protein can't be stored by the body. You have to have a fresh supply every day. The average person needs one gram of protein daily for each two pounds of body weight. So if you weigh 160 pounds, your body needs 80 grams of protein in each 24-hour period just to maintain existing muscle mass. If it doesn't get it, you risk a protein deficiency and all the myriad health problems that can go with it. Both health-wise and appearance-wise, you also make yourself susceptible to the deterioration associated with aging. Meanwhile, if you're trying to add muscle mass through exercise, your body's demand for protein increases by 100 or 200 percent, to a full gram of protein – or even a gram and a half – per pound of body weight.

Many foods supply some proteins, but those found in most vegetables are "incomplete," meaning they provide only part of the essential amino acids needed for growth, energy and health. Beans, rice and corn are all good sources of protein, for example, but they must be eaten in combination with each other or with small amounts of meat for the protein to be "complete."

(The typical Mexican peasant diet is a good example of how this works. Corn tortillas served with beans and rice provide complete protein, but only when eaten together. Eaten separately, the protein contained in corn, beans and rice is incomplete and much less beneficial than when these foods are combined.)

The most complete, highest-quality proteins come from animal foods. Unfortunately, as you recall, this is also where most saturated fat and cholesterol comes from. Much of the world suffers from a critical shortage of animal protein. But ironically the people of these protein-deficient areas don't have nearly as much heart and artery disease as we well-fed Americans do. That's because they don't eat much saturated fat, either, and get most of their calories from fruits, vegetables and whole grains.

Up until very recently, anyone who ate large amounts of animal protein was also likely to be eating large amounts of animal fat. I remember years ago when I used to eat a lot of whole-egg cheese omelets with the idea that they were supplying me with generous amounts of protein. What I didn't realize at the time was that they were also packed with saturated fat — more fat grams, in fact, than protein grams. They were a big factor in sending my cholesterol level up to around 270. But fortunately, I figured out what the problem was and took steps to correct it. Now my cholesterol is an enviable 140 — lower than that of most people half my age.

With modern production and processing techniques, animal protein and saturated fat are no longer inseparably linked. Skim milk has all the protein of whole milk, but none of the fat. Boneless, skinless chicken breasts provide just as much protein as regular chicken, but with up to 98 percent of the visible fat removed. Sliced white turkey is virtually fat-free, but all the protein is retained. An increasing variety of non-fat, high-protein cheeses is available. I don't eat it myself, but even ham now comes in a 97-percent fat-free version.

Today's Greatest Bargain

American consumers are also gradually learning the wisdom of discarding the high-fat, high-cholesterol portions of the foods they buy. Throwing away chicken and turkey skin, pork rinds and the fat trimmed from beefsteak is no more wasteful than refusing to eat orange peels or apple cores. It's the only sensible thing to do.

Some enlightened folks also realize that eggs are still an excellent buy, even when the yolks are dumped down the garbage disposer and only the whites are used. Eggs have taken a lot of bad raps from health authorities in recent years, but it's really unfair. Almost all the fat and cholesterol in an egg is in the yolk, but there's plenty of protein in the white portion to justify discarding the yolk and keeping eggs on your shopping list. Eggs are the only food I can think of that costs no more today than it did 40 or 50 years ago. I think they represent the greatest bargain in today's supermarket.

Fresh egg whites make a perfect omelet and are ideal for any recipe containing whole eggs. Simply double the number of eggs called for. The only difference is that they're white, not yellow, and their taste and texture are far superior to commercial egg substitutes. As an added bonus, eggs — and an egg separator — also provide a perfect example of how to get rid of the animal fat and keep the animal protein.

Eggs are a primary source of protein for me. I eat at least

two dozen egg whites a day. Without them, I couldn't maintain the high-intensity bodybuilding program that's part of my daily routine.

Eating for Life and Energy

I want to take a moment here to discuss my own personal approach to nutrition. Over a period of many years, I've perfected a diet that works perfectly for me and is ideally suited for my own particular lifestyle. While I doubt that you'll want to adopt it for your own use in its entirety, you may find it a valuable guide in improving your own nutrition.

I really don't like to use the word "diet" because it has some very negative connotations in many people's minds. But when I refer to my "diet," it simply means the foods I eat on a regular basis, the foods I rely on for health and energy. I don't consider myself to be "on a diet," and I don't want you to think of it in that way, either. What we're talking about is making a permanent change in our eating habits and patterns in order to get more energy and zest for life out of the foods we eat while also taking in less fat, less sugar, less sodium and fewer calories.

Let's take a look at how I typically begin my day from a nutritional standpoint:

I usually start the morning with a frothy, delicious concoction made with a dozen egg whites, two cups of frozen strawberries and a couple of packets of non-caloric sweetener. I microwave the egg whites 40 seconds, then toss them into a blender and blend at high speed until they thicken, then add the strawberries and sweetener, blend again for a few seconds and it's ready to drink.

Or I may have my eggwhites scrambled or in an omelet with mushrooms, shrimp or some other tasty addition, using non-fat Pam instead of oil or butter, and substitute a grapefruit for the strawberries.

To complete my breakfast, I have a large bowl of oatmeal with non-fat butter flavoring. The oatmeal and fruit provide the vital carbohydrates that everybody needs for short-term energy. Meanwhile, the egg whites give me a big "charge" of longer-lasting protein energy.

My hunger is totally satisfied. I feel great. I'm ready to tackle the day. I've had about 35 grams of protein, yet I've eaten only three or four grams of fat.

The Breakfast "Killer"

Now let's stop and compare my morning meal with what most people have for breakfast. A typical "big breakfast eater" is likely to have one or two whole eggs, usually cooked in grease; three or four strips of bacon; a couple of slices of buttered toast with jelly, a glass of juice, and coffee with cream and sugar.

In the process, he or she has obtained only about 20 grams of protein, compared to my 35. But the real "killer" is the amount of fat this type of breakfast contains – over 40 grams all told (almost all of it the saturated variety). Remember, that's more fat than I eat in a whole day, and this person has just finished breakfast!

At the other extreme, of course, is the person who eats nothing for breakfast. Millions of Americans fall into the category of "breakfast skippers." No breakfast at all is probably less harmful than the kind of high-fat breakfast I just described. But depriving yourself of protein and other essential nutrients is no way to start the day – not if you expect it to be a fulfilling, rewarding one.

People whose "breakfast" consists of coffee alone or coffee with doughnuts or other types of sweets that derive most of their calories from simple sugars invariably suffer from low blood sugar within an hour or so. They become progressively more grouchy, moody, irritable, sluggish and depressed as the morning wears on. By noon, they feel physically exhausted and mentally "out of it," but in most cases there's absolutely nothing wrong that a little protein and some complex carbohydrates won't cure.

(To understand how this works, think of the human body as a fireplace and the various nutritional elements as different kinds of fuel. Simple sugars are like newspaper. They burn up in one quick burst. The carbohydrates found in fresh fruits can be compared to small twigs, and the complex carbohydrates in potatoes, pasta and rice are like larger kindling. These also burn fast, but much more slowly than sugars. Protein and fats are like heavy logs. They take a long time to burn, so they provide energy for sustained periods.)

My lunch may be a sandwich of fat-free whole-grain bread piled with sliced roast turkey breast and dressed up with lettuce, tomato, mustard and non-fat mayonnaise. Or it may be fish or chicken grilled without oil and served with a salad with vinegar dressing or steamed vegetables and some type of complex carbohydrate.

At mid-morning and mid-afternoon, I have small supplemental meals. Often, when I'm in a hurry, these may consist of a powdered high-protein food replacement that can be mixed quickly in a blender with ice and water. The result is a good-tasting drink with 46 grams of protein. If I have plenty of time, I may have something more elaborate.

Potatoes Are A-OK

For dinner, I usually have chicken, fish or other seafood, and occasionally a hamburger patty made from beef round with all visible fat removed. I also have some mixed steamed vegetables and one of my all-time favorites – a big baked potato (or maybe even two). The only thing I use on my potatoes is a new product called "I Can't Believe It's Not Butter," which comes in a plastic spray bottle and can be found in the dairy case of most supermarkets. Be sure to read the label carefully and get the fat-free product. Marketed under the same name and in a very similar container is a product that contains 70 percent vegetable oil.

The fat-free version of this product is an outstanding example of the many small miracles being created by modern food technology and research. This spray tastes and looks amazingly similar to real melted butter. The big difference is that it contains no fat. There are several similar products on the market, but I like this one best.

And speaking of potatoes, let me digress for a moment. Potatoes are another wonderful natural food that have gotten an undeserved bad reputation for being fattening. Actually, nothing could be further from the truth. A medium baked or boiled potato, without anything added, has only about 100 calories and barely a trace of fat. It supplies some protein and is a great source of complex carbohydrates.

Boneless, skinless chicken breasts, by the way, can be grilled just like sirloin steaks, without any added oil, although they're 98 percent free of visible fat. In my opinion, they taste just as good, and they're even higher in protein than sirloin. I prefer mine plain, but you can add almost any kind of spices or non-fat flavorings (soy sauce, lemon or lime juice, barbecue sauce, fat-free Italian dressing, etc.) for your own special taste preference.

One reliable way to judge the fat content of seafood is by its color. In general, white fish such as sea bass, red snapper, mahi-mahi, sole, cod, flounder, perch and trout, are much lower in fat that darker fish such as salmon, most tuna and swordfish. I like sea bass so much that I buy it 50 pounds at a time for cooking at home.

White seafood, including lobster, shrimp and scallops, is universally recommended for people who want to limit their intake of dietary fat. But assuming that all seafood is automatically low in fat is a big mistake. Three ounces of steamed shrimp has only one gram of fat, for example, whereas the same amount of canned mackerel has nine times that much. It's what's added to seafood that often sends the fat content skyrocketing. A whole medium lobster has only two grams of fat, but if you dip each bite in drawn butter, chances are you'll end up eating 10 times that much fat. And canned tuna packed in oil has three times the fat of water-packed tuna. The fat content of the same brand and type of canned tuna may even vary, depending on when and where it was caught. You'll never know unless you take a moment to check the label on the can.

Score One for Consumers

This brings me to another extremely important point – and to another big advantage that today's consumer enjoys over the consumers of just yesterday in selecting healthful, nutritious, low-fat foods.

The federal government does a lot of things that irritate and anger me, but once in a while, I have to "give the devil his due." One of the best federal laws ever passed is the recent one requiring all canned or pre-packaged food items to be clearly and uniformly labeled as to their nutritional content. Score one for Uncle Sam – and score one for the health-conscious consumer, too.

The new nutrition labels show exactly how many calories and how much fat, sodium, protein and carbohydrates are in an "average serving" of the product inside the can, jar, bottle or package. The labels also clearly state how many of the calories are derived from fat. This is real progress, although it's still harder than it should be to understand all the percentages and numbers involved.

Every grocery shopper should make a habit of reading the labels. What you see on them will likely shock you at first, but it will also educate you. You'll learn, for example, that of the 100 calories in a typical frankfurter, 90 of them come from fat. And yet you'll also discover that there are now low-fat weiners and franks on the market that are 97 percent fat-free and which derive only 15-20 percent of their calories from fat.

I think you'll be amazed at the number of labels you encounter that read "Calories from Fat 0, Total Fat 0, Saturated Fat 0, Cholesterol 0."

And unlike the "old days" of just a couple of years ago, food processors and packagers can no longer use such misleading terms as "Lite" or "Reduced-Fat" or "No Cholesterol" to dupe consumers into thinking they're buying true low-fat products when they aren't. The new labels are uniform and they don't lie. They're forcing the food industry to offer us real, clear-cut choices in what we buy and eat.

Sure, You Can Afford It!

Regardless of what you may think, "eating healthy" is not an expensive luxury. If anything, it costs significantly less than the high-fat, high-sodium, high-calorie "killer" diet followed by tens of millions of Americans. This is especially true when you consider how much money you'll save on medical and hospital bills by adopting a healthier nutritional lifestyle.

In all likelihood, you may actually see your grocery bills go down, rather than up, when you start "eating healthy." You can buy a 10-pound bag of potatoes for the price of one 12-ounce bag of potato chips.

There are many other examples, too. How much does a dash of lemon juice or vinegar cost in comparison to a dollop of high-fat salad dressing? Apples and bananas are cheaper by far than Twinkies and brownies. Ounce for ounce, frozen orange juice is much more affordable than six-packs of Coke or Pepsi. In terms of the amount of vital nutrients you get for your money, fatty, salty, sugary, over-processed foods always cost more than fresh, natural ones.

As we've already mentioned, eggs are almost ridiculously inexpensive when compared to other sources of animal protein. Fresh fish and fowl cost less per pound on the average than fresh beef, pork and lamb, and frozen fish is even cheaper. Even skinless, boneless chicken breasts routinely cost less than half what you'd pay for T-bone or ribeye steak.

So stop kidding yourself about the high cost of eating right. Like so much of what we've been led to believe, it's just another myth.

What About Dining Out?

For someone who's trying to keep dietary fat to a minimum, eating out in a restaurant can pose serious problems. But, again, the situation isn't nearly as bad as it used to be.

Personally, I have three or four favorite restaurants where I've made a point of getting acquainted with the management and staff and letting them know the type of food I want. For the most part, I find restaurant people considerate and understanding about such things. If they aren't, I simply don't go back.

I'm especially fond of Chinese food. I like the taste, the emphasis on freshness and the fact that this type of ethnic fare is among the most healthful to be found in mainstream restaurants – so long as it isn't too "westernized." At my favorite Chinese restaurant, I often ask the chef to make up a dish with shrimps, scallops, white chicken and chinese vegetables. By ordering steamed rice, rather than fried, and steering clear of the soy sauce and fried noodles, I get a great meal that's near perfect from a nutritional standpoint.

Most restaurants – even those that feature high-fat specialties – offer a few low-fat options. And, increasingly, they even set aside one section of their menu for lower-fat, lower-calorie selections. In Texas, for example, where fajitas are one of the most popular entrees around, a number of restaurants now offer fajitas grilled without oil and served without such high-fat accompaniments as guacamolé and sour cream.

Even most fast-food places now feature salad bars with one or two types of fat-free dressings. The trick here, in addition to avoiding regular salad dressings, is to steer clear of such fat-laden "fixin's" as grated cheese, diced luncheon meat, those imitation bacon bits, buttery croutons, olives (another veggie that's almost all fat calories), and pasta and potato salads made with regular mayonnaise.

Another viable option is to "brown-bag it." Millions of students and workers do this every day. But instead of the usual fare of peanut butter or salami sandwiches, chips and cookies, bring your favorite low-fat foods. I do this frequently, not only when I'm going to the office, but when I'm travelling. Whenever

I fly commercially, I take a sandwich along and avoid that notorious airline food. And when I go somewhere like Paris, where everything seems to be swimming in rich sauces, I take along a bagful of healthful food in plastic containers packed in dry ice.

Four Simple Rules

Admittedly, I'm more stringent about my diet than 99.9 percent of the people I meet. I also have the good fortune to be able to eat and enjoy the same basic foods over and over without getting burned out on them. You may need more variety in your meals, and you may find it hard to stick to the same strict criteria I use.

But the point is, you don't have to follow a regimen like mine. You can easily adapt the simple guiding principles I use to your own particular needs and preferences. The rules are simple. They really come down to just four things:

(1) Cut down on the amount of fat you eat – to 30 percent or less of your total calorie consumption – and make a point of knowing how much fat your food contains. Recognizing the enemy is half the battle.

(2) Make sure you get plenty of protein – one gram a day for each two pounds of body weight – with emphasis on such low-fat animal sources as lean meat and fish, egg whites and fat-free dairy products.

(3) Fill up on complex carbohydrates – fresh fruits and vegetables, potatoes, rice, pasta (without the garlic butter or cream sauce), whole-grain breads – and minimize your use of simple sugars.

(4) Don't add salt to your food and beware of the excess sodium contained in salted chips, pickles and many other snack foods (too much sodium can raise your blood pressure and damage your kidneys), and drink plenty of water.

It's OK to indulge in a special treat once in a while, especially when there are so many fat-free, healthful treats to choose from. Even I can't resist an occasional dish of non-fat frozen yogurt. Once in a while, I even have a vegetable pizza made with fat-free mozzarella cheese. If you want to have a steak now and then, have a steak. It's not what you eat every week or two that determines how healthy, attractive and long-lived you are – it's what you eat every day.

No More "Dieting"

...adopt a new, healthier nutritional lifestyle, it can ... "dieting" forever. Never again will you have to ... those diet-drink concoctions for lunch and suf-...gs all afternoon. You can forget about living on "rabbit food" and never having a hearty meal.

Remember, your goal isn't to "reduce" or lose weight – not anymore. If you're very much overweight, that weight loss will invariably come. But your goal is to look better, feel better and live a longer, fuller life.

If you want to use nutrition effectively to lengthen and enhance your life, improve your appearance and protect your health, eating wisely has to become part of your everyday routine. But you don't have to deprive yourself. You don't have to starve yourself or endure endless hunger. In fact, when you eat five times a day the way I do, it's almost impossible to be hungry.

If you're hungry, eat! But eat something that's good for you. The trick is to get the maximum amount of protein and complex carbohydrates with a minimum of calories and fat. That's really the only trick there is. If you can do that, you've got it made nutritionally.

To give you some general guidance on how to get the kind of healthy nutrition that suits your particular needs, I'm including samples of four different daily menus at the end of this chapter. They start with a 1,500-calorie version, which is about what a moderately active woman of average build should consume in a day. From there, they go on to 2,000-calorie and 2,500-calorie versions, which supply sufficient "fuel" for most active men. Very few people need more than 2,500 calories daily, but to meet all the nutritional needs of those who follow a really rigorous physical training program similar to mine, the calorie count can be increased to as much as 3,000 per day by proportionately increasing the amount of protein and carbohydrates shown.

If you want other ideas on how to keep your menus varied, nutritionally adequate and interesting while limiting fat and calories, go to your library. There are dozens of cookbooks today that offer low-fat or no-fat recipes. One of the best is the American Heart Association's *Low-Fat, Low-Cholesterol Cookbook*. You'll be amazed at how good some of these dishes taste and how hunger-satisfying they are.

Within a short time, eating for good health, disease prevention and maximum vitality during your second 50 years can become an integral part of your daily routine – something you do automatically without having to think about it before every meal. Within as little as two weeks, you can take major steps to re-educate your tastes and readjust your eating habits. In effect, you can start a new life.

I hope you'll try it for two weeks and see what happens.

Just two weeks from today, I predict you'll be able to see exciting results in yourself. You'll see them in the mirror, on the bathroom scales, in the way your clothes fit. But you'll also feel these results deep inside yourself. You'll experience a sense of wellbeing, a sense of satisfaction and being in control of your life that you may never have known before.

And the last thing in the world you'll want to do is go back to being the way you were before. I guarantee it.

SAMPLE HIGH-PROTEIN, LOW-FAT MENUS

1,500 CALORIES

	Calories	Protein (g)	Fat (g)	Carbohydrates (g)
BREAKFAST:				
8 egg whites	160	26	–	2
12 oz. melon (honeydew or cantaloupe)	120	2	–	26
Totals	280	28	–	28
LUNCH:				
6 oz. fish	180	36	2	–
lettuce, tomato	50	–	–	11
1 cooked yam (8 oz.)	220	5	–	48
Totals	450	41	2	59
P.M. SNACK:				
1 cup applesauce	110	–	–	28
2/3 cup oats				
Totals	310	10	4	64

DINNER:

4 oz. fish	125	21	1	–
1/2 lb. steamed veggies	160	4	–	16
1 cup rice	180	4	1	41
Totals	465	29	2	57

(8–10 glasses of water throughout day; limit of 2 caffeinated diet beverages per day)

TOTAL FOR DAY	**1,505**	**108**	**8**	**230**

2,000 CALORIES

	Calories	Protein (g)	Fat (g)	Carbohydrates (g)
BREAKFAST:				
10 egg whites	200	33	–	2
1/2 medium potato	60	1	–	37
2 cups fresh fruit	120	1	–	28
Totals	380	35	–	67
A.M. SNACK:				
1 large apple	100	–	–	26
LUNCH:				
1 can (6.5-oz) tuna	205	40	4	–
2 pickle slices,				
1 small tomato	50	–	–	11
1 cooked yam (8 oz.)	220	5	–	48
Totals	475	45	–	59
P.M. SNACK:				
6 egg whites	120	19	–	–
1/2 cup rice	90	2	–	20
1/4 cup veggies	25	1	–	4
Totals	235	22	–	24

POSTWORKOUT:

	Calories	Protein	Fat	Carbs
1 cup applesauce	110	–	–	28
1/3 cup oats	100	5	2	18
Totals	210	5	2	46

DINNER:

	Calories	Protein	Fat	Carbs
1/2 lb. fish	225	40	2	–
3/4 cup steamed veggies	75	–	–	19
1 cup rice	180	4	1	41
Totals	480	44	3	60

(8–10 glasses of water throughout day; limit of 2 non–caloric caffeine drinks per day)

TOTAL FOR DAY	**2095**	**151**	**9**	**284**

2,500 CALORIES

	Calories	Protein (g)	Fat (g)	Carbohydrates (g)

BREAKFAST:

	Calories	Protein	Fat	Carbs
10 egg whites	200	33	–	2
1 large potato	235	1	–	37
2 cups fruit	120	1	–	28
Totals	555	35	–	67

A.M. SNACK:

	Calories	Protein	Fat	Carbs
1 banana	110	–	–	28
1/3 cup oats	100	5	2	18
1/2 cup applesauce	55	–	–	14
Totals	265	5	2	60

LUNCH:

	Calories	Protein	Fat	Carbs
1 can tuna (6.5 o	205	40	–	–
2 pickle slices, 1 small tomato	50	–	–	11
1 cooked yam (8 oz.)	220	5	–	48
Totals	465	45	–	59

P.M. SNACK:

4 oz. chicken	140	22	3	–
1 cup rice	180	4	1	41
1/4 cup veggies	25	1	–	4
Totals	345	27	4	45

POSTWORKOUT:

1 cup applesauce	110	–	–	28
2/3 cup oats	200	10	4	36
Totals	310	10	4	64

DINNER:

1/2 lb. chicken or fish	300	45	6	–
3/4 cup steamed veggies	75	–	–	19
1 cup rice	180	4	1	41
Totals	505	49	7	60

(8-10 glasses of water throughout day; limit of 2 non-caloric caffeine drinks per day)

TOTAL FOR DAY	**2445**	**171**	**17**	**354**

> "Every man desires to live long, but
> no man would be old."
> –JONATHAN SWIFT

CHAPTER 5

Life-Saving and Life-Stretching Supplements

Almost 50 years ago, I became one of a mere handful of Americans who took vitamin supplements religiously every day. Back then, in the late '40s and early '50s, it was universally assumed that if you ate "three square meals a day," you automatically got all the vitamins you needed.

Except for sickly children, who were sometimes given vitamins on the advice of their doctors, people who took them every day were considered eccentric at best and downright nutty at worst. Some vitamins that we take for granted today, such as Vitamin E, had only been identified for a few years and weren't readily available for public consumption even if the public had wanted them. Scientists themselves didn't understand very much about vitamins and minerals or the myriad effects they have on the human body.

No one knew, for example, that Vitamin C was a powerful infection fighter. No one realized that osteoporosis – the brittle-bones disease that affects so many older women – was directly related to long-term deficiencies of calcium and Vitamin D. No one had any idea that Vitamin E could prevent scarring in wounds, much less that it and other nutritional elements with anti-oxidant properties, such as beta carotene, would be used in the 1990s to prevent coronary heart disease.

I didn't know anything about vitamins, either, of course. But I started taking them because I wanted to do everything I could possibly do to build up my body and improve my physical strength and stamina. If vitamins would give me an edge over other guys in my struggle to climb the ladder of success, that was all the motivation I needed to give them a try. Most of the people I knew at the time would've laughed at the idea, and a lot of them did laugh, but I didn't care. I was determined to give myself every advantage possible.

Today, close to a half-century later, I'm still taking large daily doses of vitamins and minerals, as well as other supplements. I've never regretted starting on a program of nutritional supplementation at an early age. I think it definitely did give me an edge – and just as importantly, I think it still does. But in contrast to the "I'll try anything that might help" approach I took as a teenager, I now structure my nutritional supplements with specific goals in mind.

It's No Joking Matter

Nobody laughs at anyone else for taking vitamins these days. Tens of millions of Americans take them routinely every day. More and more doctors are recommending vitamins to their patients, instead of telling them, as they once did, that if you eat a well-balanced diet, vitamins are unnecessary.

Meanwhile, science is producing additional proof every year that taking various nutritional elements in doses far larger than any amount of food could possibly supply can be a key health factor – both in helping us fight off disease or injury when it strikes and in preventing it in the first place. Nothing has captured more public attention recently than the strong evidence, developed in dozens of studies, that large daily doses of Vitamin E, Vitamin C and beta carotene can stop hardening of the arteries before it occurs by protecting artery walls against cholesterol deposits.

If anything, vitamins may have become too popular with the public – at least as far as some powerful forces in our society are concerned. There have been determined efforts within the past few years on the part of the FDA and the AMA to persuade Congress to pass laws that would sharply restrict the availability and use of vitamins by the American people.

These forces would like to see vitamin supplements classified as prescription drugs and make them available only with a doctor's prescription. They haven't yet succeeded in this shameful attempt to abridge citizens' rights, thank God, but I'm sure they haven't given up in their efforts, either. This is just one example of how seriously the vitamin issue is being taken today.

The Pace Accelerates

At first, our knowledge of the relationship between certain nutritional elements and the prevention and cure of specific diseases developed very slowly. Only a century or two has passed, for example, since we discovered that iodine prevented goiter and that the Vitamin C in citrus fruits prevented scurvy. But now the pace of learning is accelerating every day.

I'm thoroughly convinced that in years to come, vitamins and other nutritional elements will be used successfully to treat and prevent all kinds of diseases. We already know that adult-onset diabetes can usually be prevented by a high-protein, low-fat, low-sugar diet alone. I believe that within the mysterious, fascinating labyrinth of nutrition lie key secrets for holding at bay such other widespread degenerative illnesses as Parkinson's Disease, Alzheimer's Disease – and even cancer.

In my opinion, we've barely scratched the surface in using vitamins to fight disease and aging. For instance, recent medical research indicates that the same destructive "oxygen free radicals" which contribute to coronary artery disease also travel through the human body to stir up trouble in other places. They are now known to be a key factor in causing cataracts, the vision-robbing growths that affect millions of Americans in their 50s, 60s and 70s.

The Fountain of Youth?

Cataracts and clogged arteries are symptoms of aging, but there are other aging symptoms linked to free radicals that aren't as easily detected. For more than 40 years, researchers have noticed that free-radical injuries accumulate in cells as people grow older, but no one knew if the damage actually caused aging or if aging merely allowed the damage to happen.

Then, in early 1994, a study at Southern Methodist University showed that when fruit flies were genetically engineered to resist free-radical damage, they lived 30 percent longer than ordinary fruit flies. This marked the first proof that free-radical damage actually causes aging.

If Vitamin E and other anti-oxidant vitamins can prevent these roaming culprits from damaging arteries, the same vitamins may also be able to prevent cataracts. Carried a step further, anti-oxidants may fight free-radical damage at the cellular level, too. Much remains to be learned, but if this is true, Vitamin E, Vitamin C and beta carotene may well prove to be key components of the Fountain of Youth.

The question is, do you want to sit around and wait for years for suppositions like this to become proven fact, or do you want to claim the health and longevity benefits that can come from taking vitamin supplements right now?

Every American past the age of 50 has a huge vested interest in seeing these secrets unlocked and the breakthroughs in nutritional research continue. But in the meantime, I think the only intelligent course is to make sure we don't fall victim to preventable diseases by utilizing the protective vitamins at our disposal today.

Unlike me, most people haven't been taking vitamins most of their lives, and in many cases they're already nutritionally deficient. For them, their 50th birthdays can represent a major crossroads. Their health can either deteriorate with alarming speed or they can use our emerging knowledge about the value of supplements to ward off disease and make themselves stronger than ever before.

Meanwhile, though, there are numerous obstacles to overcome if we are to get maximum benefit from the vitamins, minerals and nutrition-based therapies that are now available.

Prevention Isn't Allowed

One of the biggest problems is the continued reluctance of both the medical hierarchy and the federal bureaucracy to approve – much less promote – the use of nutritional elements for maintaining health and preventing disease. Even in the face of overwhelming evidence that these elements work, the resistance to their use goes on. Part of this relates back to the idea we discussed earlier – that the whole focus of the nation's medical

Life-Saving & Life-Stretching Supplements

establishment is treating existing illnesses, not preventing them before they happen.

U.S. pharmaceutical companies, for instance, aren't allowed by the FDA to market and distribute products to prevent disease, only those used to treat it once it develops. Under our present laws, the only drugs the FDA can approve are those designed to counteract specific disorders or disease conditions. Thus, these companies have little or no incentive to conduct expensive research into preventatives.

It's as if keeping people healthy to begin with is totally unimportant and immaterial. How ridiculous can you get? And how dangerous would it be if the FDA were able to exercise the same kind of arbitrary, autocratic rule over vitamins, minerals and other nutritional supplements as it does over prescription drugs?

Carried to extremes (as is so often the case with the government), you wouldn't be allowed to take an anti-oxidant vitamin to prevent atherosclerosis until after you'd already had a heart attack. That really makes a lot of sense, doesn't it?

Are Vitamins "Toxic"?

Another problem is the misinformation that is still being circulated about vitamins – much of it intentional. There are persistent reports that large doses of vitamins can be "toxic." Although there's never been a documented case of serious illness associated with a vitamin overdose, the rumors and rumblings continue. It's perfectly true that mega-doses of vitamins can cause occasional unwanted side effects. For instance, some people have gotten diarrhea after taking 30,000-40,000 units of Vitamin C in a 24-hour period.

But "toxic"? When we compare any documented side effects from vitamins to all the truly dangerous toxic substances in our lives – nuclear wastes, polluted air, acid rain, poisoned soil, heavy metals in our food chain, known carcinogens in our drinking water, etc. – the minuscule risk associated with vitamins is almost laughable.

Just a few years ago, the medical and governmental "control freaks" wanted to limit the potency of individual vitamin tablets. Individual capsules of Vitamin A would have been limited to a maximum of 20,000 units each to avoid potential toxicity. Yet three chicken livers contain more than 32,000 units of Vitamin A,

just as much sense – or as little – to limit the
livers one person may eat in a day.
out vitamin toxicity is just another part of a
ned to keep the public wary and uncertain
..uonal supplements are concerned. The point is,
..ere's no real need for anyone to consume the volume of vitamins theoretically required to produce toxicity. But there is a need for everyone – especially everyone over age 50 – to take vitamin supplements in effective dosages every day.

Food Alone Isn't Enough

It's simply impossible to obtain all, or even most, of the vitamins and minerals necessary for disease prevention from the food we eat. This is particularly true if most of our food is overprocessed and cooked at high temperatures. Deep frying, as practiced in thousands of fast-food restaurants, spells death for many key vitamins.

But even when we choose the most healthful foods and prepare them in the least damaging way, they just aren't able to provide all the vitamins we need. Unlike Vitamin A, which occurs in liberal quantities in dozens of different meats, dairy products, vegetables and fruits, other vitamins essential to preserving health and preventing disease are much less plentiful in food.

For instance, to get my daily dose of 2,000 units of Vitamin C from "natural sources" instead of one small pill, I'd have to eat about 27 medium oranges or 15 average-size grapefruit. To get my 1,000 daily units of Vitamin E from food would be out of the question, since E is found only in the oil of whole grains and nuts. Wheat germ is the only really valuable source that isn't extremely high in fat.

Studies at the University of Texas Southwestern Medical School show that a minimum daily dosage of 400 units of Vitamin E is necessary to prevent the oxidation of cholesterol in the bloodstream, which leads to potentially deadly lesions in artery walls. But trying to obtain even this much E from foods is totally impractical, if not impossible. The only feasible solution is to swallow one or more 400-unit gelatin capsules each day at a cost of just over a dime apiece. That's an incredibly small price to pay for heart attack prevention.

One final note about Vitamin E: Although it costs slightly more, it's important to be sure you're taking the variety of E

Life-Saving & Life-Stretching Supplement

composed of "d-alpha tocopherols," not "dl-alpha" tocopherols." Without going into a lot of technical alpha" variety is simply higher quality and more effective than the other types.

My Own "Miracle Cure"

Natural Vitamin D, the so-called "sunshine vitamin," is almost non-existent in food. Artificially produced Vitamin D is added to milk in an effort to ensure that children get a sufficient supply. But the only edible substances in which this vitamin occurs naturally in any quantity is fish-liver oil – especially cod-liver oil.

To illustrate the tremendous effect that a specific nutritional element or combination of elements can have on a specific health problem, I want to tell you a story about cod-liver oil.

When I was still in my 30s, I developed severe pains and swelling in my joints. The discomfort went on for weeks, and I finally went to a doctor, who examined me and diagnosed my condition as rheumatoid arthritis, possibly brought on by joint damage I had suffered as a wrestler, plus the stresses of intensive weight training.

I was stunned and unnerved. Arthritis was not only a notorious crippler, it was also an "old person's disease." I was too young and healthy to be sidelined by something like that, but the doctor was sure of his diagnosis. He suggested surgery to relieve the condition.

While I was still trying to decide what to do, someone told me about a book written by Dr. Dale Alexander entitled *Arthritis and Common Sense*. The book recommended taking several doses of cod-liver oil daily, so I bought some and tried it. I was absolutely amazed. Within two weeks, all the pain and swelling were gone.

I continued taking cod-liver oil for about two years, then discontinued it. But in all the years since, I've never had another symptom of arthritis. Several times over the years, I've mentioned my experience with this "miracle cure" to other physicians. They've invariably shrugged it off as some sort of lucky coincidence.

Was it the Vitamin D in the cod-liver oil that cured me? Or was it something else? To this day, I don't have an answer to this question, yet I'm 100 percent convinced that something in the cod-liver oil permanently ended my arthritis. And if it should ever come back, I guarantee you the first thing I'll do is start taking cod-liver oil again!

This story illustrates how relatively little we know, even today, about certain vitamins. Medical science continues to operate under the basic assumption that only children need Vitamin D. However, it is known that when sufficient doses of Vitamin D and calcium are continued into adulthood, they can prevent osteoporosis (porous bones) in post-menopausal women.

Since arthritis is also a disease of the joints and bones, could something as simple as a few teaspoons of cod-liver oil each day protect you from this crippling disease that now rages through our over-50 population in epidemic proportions? There's one sure way to find out.

Getting Enough Fiber

One of the most important ingredients of overall nutritional health actually has no nutritive value at all. Yet this substance is absolutely essential to efficient digestion and elimination, and it's the most effective preventative known against intestinal cancer. It isn't protein, carbohydrate or fat, and it doesn't add a single calorie to your diet, but you need it every day.

I'm talking about fiber, of course. Some people call it "roughage" or "dietary bulk." All these terms mean the same thing.

Fiber occurs naturally in practically all fruits, vegetables and whole grains. But most of the refined and over-processed foods typically eaten by Americans today are terribly deficient in fiber. Such wholesome, health-building foods as meat, fish, eggs and dairy products also contain no fiber. Consequently, millions of us don't get enough fiber in our daily diet.

The foods with the highest concentrations of fiber include broccoli, carrots, leafy green vegetables, oatmeal, brown rice, corn, whole-grain bread, etc. Wheat bran is especially rich in fiber. The vast majority of us don't eat enough of these foods. When we don't, the lack of bulk in our diet can not only cause problems with irregularity, but also sharply increase our risk of colon cancer.

If you're like me and don't particularly like broccoli or some of these other foods, there's a simple solution to the problem.

Just as I take supplemental protein to keep my body ready for rigorous physical training, I also take a fiber supplement every day to prevent problems before they start. the wise thing to do is take a high-fiber supplement every day.

Personally, I like Metamucil and Konsyl. By combining these two, I get all the benefits of natural fiber in a convenient, good-tasting form. There are several good fiber supplements on the market, so there's no reason not to get the fiber you need.

Let the Buyer Beware

Unfortunately, there are also a lot of low-quality nutritional supplements being marketed today. Many of the products that line the vitamin counters of drugstores and supermarkets are, in fact, virtually worthless. And even more unfortunately, these are the very products that most people buy and use, because they're the most widely advertised and have the highest visibility.

The average person has been sold on the idea that taking one of the so-called "high-potency multi-vitamin" pills once a day will supply everything he or she needs. Actually, nothing could be further from the truth. The fact is, many of these all-inclusive, once-a-day formulations contain such small amounts of such substandard and synthetic vitamins that you might as well be swallowing an M&M.

I've been buying – and selling – multiple vitamin tablets for decades. Clare and I used to market our own brand of vitamin tablets in our health clubs. As a result, I consider myself as knowledgeable as anyone in America on the subject of multiple vitamins. When I choose a particular tablet, I check the contents carefully and make sure they're all there in sufficient quantity and quality. You should, too.

The multiple vitamin I take contains 25,000 units of A, all the essential minerals and all the B-complex vitamins (B-1, B-2, B-6, B-12, niacinamide, folic acid and pantothenic acid). Many good multi-vitamins also contain some C and E, but in order to get sufficient amounts of these vitamins, it's necessary to take them separately.

In addition, I take three 100-milligram tablets of B-1 (or thiamine) daily, which I believe is especially important. Deficiencies of B-1 are associated with a variety of ailments, ranging from constipation to mental depression and fatigue to heart disease. I also take an injection of B-12 once a week, since I don't eat much of the foods that supply it most abundantly, such as cheese, milk, egg yolks and liver. Deficiencies of B-12 can cause anemia, nervousness and spinal cord damage.

They Aren't "Pep Pills"

Lots of people are disappointed when they start taking vitamins for the first time, but this is generally because they expect the wrong things from the vitamins they take. Despite what you may have been led to believe, vitamins won't give you bursts of extra pep and vigor. They aren't supposed to. The protein, carbohydrates and fat in your diet are the elements that supply you with energy. Vitamins serve another function entirely. Their role is to keep the human machine functioning efficiently, rebuilding the damage we all inflict on it, and warding off the disease processes that threaten it.

Anytime you're deficient in vitamins or minerals, you open the door to illness and the ravages of aging. If you want to keep that door closed and locked, take supplements.

Do I feel "different" because of the supplements I take? I can't honestly say that I do – not consciously, anyway. Of course, after nearly 50 years of taking vitamins every day, I wouldn't be likely to notice a difference, anyway.

On the other hand, I do credit vitamins with helping me maintain the kind of overall health, strength and stamina I want. I don't think I'd be nearly as healthy or vigorous today if I hadn't followed a faithful vitamin regimen over all these years. But even if you've never taken supplements on a regular basis, it's never too late to start, and the benefits to your health will begin almost immediately.

Vitamin and mineral supplements have helped make it possible for me to do things that many people half my age can't do. I have no doubt that they've helped keep me free of disease and contributed to my remarkable ability to recover from injuries. I'm equally confident that they'll continue to give me a vital edge in the years ahead.

In short, I'm no more likely to quit taking nutritional supplements than I am to quit eating.

> "Since the body tends to deteriorate more quickly with age, the effect that bodybuilding has in building, shaping and strengthening the body is even more pronounced in older bodybuilders than in younger ones. "'Am I too old to do bodybuilding?' I am frequently asked. My answer is always, 'You're too old not to.'"
> —ARNOLD SCHWARZENEGGER

CHAPTER 6

Exercise and Fitness— Why It's Easier Than You Think

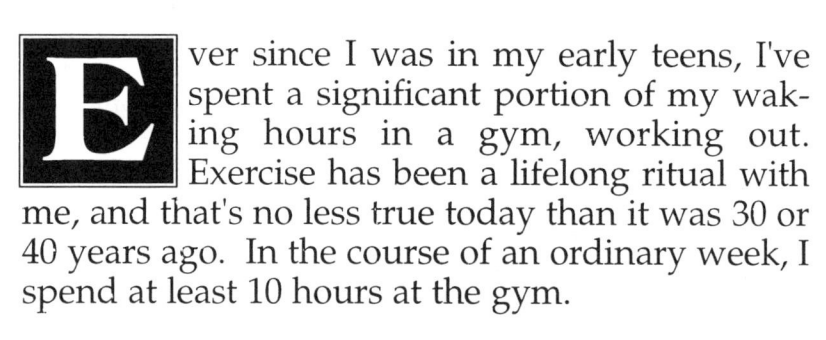

Ever since I was in my early teens, I've spent a significant portion of my waking hours in a gym, working out. Exercise has been a lifelong ritual with me, and that's no less true today than it was 30 or 40 years ago. In the course of an ordinary week, I spend at least 10 hours at the gym.

Because of this, many people naturally assume that I'm some sort of exercise freak who just loves to sweat and strain on a weight machine or a treadmill. In reality, though, nothing could be further from the truth. Sometimes, when I'm tired after a long day, it's all I can do to force myself to go to the gym for a two-hour workout. All I want to do is relax. In that respect, I'm no different from anybody else. I don't love exercise, but I do love the results. I like being stronger, more fit and better built at 62 than most 22-year-olds are. The drive to be the best I can be is what prompted me to start exercising in the first place. It's what has kept me exercising all these years, and it's what will motivate me to keep right on exercising as long as I live.

Make no mistake, though – exercise can be enjoyable and often is. The idea that every minute spent working out has to be sheer agony is as wrong as it can be. Unless you're training at an intense, competitive level, you can forget that outdated philosophy of "no pain, no gain." Thanks to modern technology and techniques, exercise today can be more comfortable and more closely suited to an individual's own personal preferences and needs than ever before.

Working out can – and should – make you feel good inside and out. Along with the feeling of satisfaction it brings, there's a natural "high" that comes from regular exercise. It's partly the physical sensation of feeling your level of fitness increase and knowing you're improving your strength, endurance, vitality and overall health. And part of it's psychological – a sense of accomplishment and gratification that comes from knowing you're doing something good for yourself.

It Started With Vanity

As a vain young man, my first objective in working out was simply to look good. I still remember looking enviously at photographs of "muscle man" John Grimek in a magazine and marvelling at the incredible physique of the man who dominated the world of bodybuilding in the '40s.

I thought, "Gee, I'd like to look like that." But unlike most guys my age, my response didn't stop there. Vanity and envy spurred me to action, and I headed for the nearest gym almost immediately. At the time, my reasons for exercising may have been pretty shallow, but those reasons have deepened and broadened over the years as I've learned more about the benefits of exercise.

Today, we know a hundred times as much about those benefits as we did when I started out. We know that cross-training, which combines aerobic exercises with weight-resistance exercises, can do a lot more than merely make you look good. Having big biceps and drawing admiring glances from the girls is nice, but those are just "fringe benefits" compared to the main atttraction. Exercise can also strengthen the most important muscle in your body – your heart. It can increase the ability of your lungs to take in oxygen and the ability of your body to use it. Practiced with enough frequency and intensity, it can make you virtually "heart attack-proof."

There's no longer the slightest doubt that we all need regular, vigorous exercise if we want to live the longest, fullest life possible. When I started working out, almost no one other than bodybuilders engaged in regular year-round exercise. Even college and professional athletes worked out sporadically or not at all in the off-season. But that was because we didn't know what we know today.

We hadn't yet come to understand that regular exercise is vital to human well-being – so vital that the American Heart Association recently added lack of exercise to its official list of major risk factors for heart disease – along with cigarette smoking, obesity, high cholesterol and high blood pressure. The key question is no longer "Should I?" It's "How?" and "When?"

So regardless of what youthful ambitions may have inspired me in the beginning, the most important thing is that I stayed with a program of regular exercise, and I've been at it ever since. Exercise is an ingrained part of my life and my lifestyle. I hope to persuade you to make it part of yours.

It can not only add youth to your appearance and years to your life, it can also add more quality and zest to those years than you may ever have dreamed possible.

In the process, it can give your vanity quite a boost, too.

The Choice Is Yours

The first thing I want to emphasize is that you don't need a lot of expensive equipment to conduct a successful exercise program. You don't necessarily need to join a health club or do your workouts in a gym, either. I, for one, enjoy going to the gym. I also dislike exercising at home. But these are personal choices that you should make for yourself.

Just because I helped pioneer the health club concept in this country doesn't mean I'm trying to sell you a health club membership. Part of my purpose in this chapter will be to tell you what I think you should look for in a health club and give you an idea of how much you should pay for membership, then let you decide if that's the best route for you.

First and foremost, the important thing is to do *something* and do it regularly. As millions of Americans have learned in recent years, simply walking is a wonderful form of exercise. The only "investment" required is the price of a good pair of shoes. It can be done just about anywhere at any time – in a park or a shopping mall, on the street where you live, even in your own yard. You can do it alone or with one or more partners.

While walking doesn't tone all your muscles, it does firm and strengthen your leg muscles. It also has valuable aerobic benefits if you walk long enough and at a fast enough pace. For many people, a regular walk of 30 to 45 minutes three or four times a week is their total exercise program. And while it falls short of being ideal, it's much, much better than nothing at all.

For others, regular walking serves as a good starting point. It allows people to establish a basic routine that can be added to and serve as a springboard for a more comprehensive ongoing exercise program.

Or, on the other hand, you can join a health club for an initial fee of $150-$200 and dues of $15-$20 a month and hire your own personal trainer to put you through your paces for $25-$50 per hour. This is the optimum approach, in my opinion. But it all depends on how much money you can afford to spend, how much equipment you like at your disposal, how highly organized a program you prefer, and whether you're a self-starter or someone who needs to be pushed a little sometimes.

In between these two opposite ends of the spectrum is an almost endless variety of individual approaches to regular exercise. You can ride a bike, stationary or real. You can jog or run in place. You can swim or dance or rollerblade. You can lift barbells or do calisthenics. You can even do yoga if you're so inclined.

To repeat: The important thing is to do *something* on a regular basis.

Sure You Have Time!

People can come up with a wide variety of excuses for not exercising, and during my years as a bodybuilder and health club operator, I think I've heard them all. But by far the most popular is "I don't have time."

I don't believe it. I don't think they really believe it, either.

No matter who you are or what kind of schedule you're on, you can find some time to exercise if you really want to. It's a matter of priorities. In my experience, the majority of people who are quickest to say "I don't have time" are the very same ones who manage to fit an extended after-work "cocktail hour" into their daily schedule. Or play a round of golf a couple of times a week. Or bowl in a league. (Golf and bowling are lots of fun, by the way, but they don't count as real exercise.) Or read a novel every week. Or take a nap before dinner. Or play cards or work crossword puzzles or go fishing or sunbathe or putter in the yard.

I'm not saying that any of these activities is unimportant, and I'm not trying to tell you what to do with your leisure time. But if you can spend three or four or five hours out of a typical week indulging in one or more of the pursuits mentioned above, you can find that same amount of time to exercise.

Again, it comes down to establishing priorities for yourself. We invariably find time for the things we consider important. If living a healthy, satisfying second 50 years is important to you, you'll stop conning yourself about not having time and make a permanent place in your life for exercise.

Make It Manageable

Look, it *doesn't take that long*. If you don't believe it, try this:

Start off with something totally manageable. Set aside just 10 or 15 minutes at least three times a week. It doesn't matter what time of day you choose. It can be morning, noontime, afternoon or evening. Pick any type of aerobic exercise you want. Ride a stationary bike while you watch TV. Take a brisk walk around the block a few times. Turn on some lively music and dance. Play tag or skip rope with your kids.

Basically, you can't go wrong by starting with simple fast walking. It's excellent aerobic exercise, which benefits your whole cardiovascular system. It can lower your blood pressure, and there's some evidence that it can even lower your cholesterol.

Whatever you do, the important thing is to keep moving, to get your cardiovascular system tuned up – your blood circulating, your heart rate accelerating, your lungs pumping air. You could wake up with some sore muscles after the first session or two, depending on how out of shape you are, but the soreness shouldn't be severe and it shouldn't last long. So don't even think about quitting. Just hang in there for three or four weeks and see what happens.

As you continue these activity sessions on a regular basis, you begin to speed up your metabolism. This means that your body burns more calories, not only when you're exercising but when you're sitting still. As a result, after a week or two, you may even discover you've lost a little weight, although you're still eating just as much as ever.

Chances are, you'll also notice some other things, too. You may experience certain subtle changes in your physical and mental state. Maybe you don't tire quite as easily as you did just a few weeks ago. Maybe there's a little more bounce in your step. Maybe you sleep a little better at night. Maybe you don't seem to get indigestion or headaches as often. Maybe you aren't quite as irritable or uptight.

What you're beginning to see are the real, tangible results of regular exercise.

Beware of "Overdoing It"

Once you feel the difference and realize what's happening, the natural tendency is to want to do more. This is good. You *should* do more than the minimum, but it's also important not to try to press too hard or go too fast. There's no need to rush it. You're in this for the long haul, remember? You have plenty of time to achieve the results you want. Meanwhile, nothing can kill an exercise program faster than injury or exhaustion caused by forcing your body to do something it isn't ready to do yet.

In a walking program that starts with 10 or 15 minutes at a time, it's best to increase the length of the sessions in increments of five minutes or less, then stay at that level for a couple of weeks – until you're comfortable with it – before increasing the length again. Once you're doing 30-45 minutes at least three or four times a week, you will have reached the level where you're producing genuine cardiovascular fitness. There's no actual need to go beyond that unless you just want to. If you feel the desire to do more, consider adding a second activity for variety.

Adding a touch of weight training to your routine, for instance, can be as simple as carrying a couple of one- or two-pound hand weights along on your walks and lifting and lowering them every few steps.

More Isn't Always Better

Among those who adopt and maintain long-term regular exercise programs, a certain percentage always seem to have a tendency to overdo it. This is especially true of people with a highly competitive nature.

Some runners who get a "high" from running five miles can be satisfied with that accomplishment, but others feel a compulsion to try for 10, or 15, or more. With some weightlifters, it becomes a macho thing to be able to bench press more than the other guy. But this is the way to hurt yourself – sometimes seriously.

Trying to lift more than you're capable of lifting can severely damage your back, shoulders, knees or other joints. Besides that, it's pointless. Achieving proper muscle tone and appearance depends more on how often you repeat an exercise and the form you use than in how much you lift. Doing at least 12 to 15 repetitions of a comfortable weight-resistance exercise will do more to help tone muscles than straining to do fewer reps at a more difficult level.

Carried to extremes, exercise can become catabolic – meaning it will actually burn up all the nutrients in the body and began devouring lean muscle mass. This is particularly true for marathon runners, who often push their bodies to the absolute limit for periods of four hours or more without rest. Most marathon runners have almost zero body fat to begin with, and in my opinion, many of them are jeopardizing their health. Several recent tragic incidents in which seemingly healthy marathon runners died suddenly and unexpectedly can almost certainly be blamed on the tremendous stresses to which they expose themselves.

Medical experts have now come to the conclusion that there definitely is such a thing as too much exercise. There's a point at which over-exercising can become just as hazardous to health as no exercise at all.

Set Realistic Limits

Whatever type of exercise you're doing, set reasonable limits for yourself. Always take time to warm up for a few minutes before you start. Increase levels gradually. And when you're tired – really tired – stop. If you experience any physical symptoms that seem unusual, check with your doctor.

I don't recommend that anyone try to follow the exercise regimen I follow – particularly anyone who's reached the age of 40 or 50 without regular workouts. For most people, an average of less than an hour of exercise four or five times a week is plenty. A good cross-training mix might include about an hour of weight-resistance exercise one day alternated with about a half-hour of cardiovascular exercise the next day. If you truly enjoy the routine and want to increase the length of your sesssions, fine. If not, you're still giving yourself 90-95 percent of the health, appearance and longevity benefits that exercise can provide.

The point is this: We don't need a nation of professional athletes or obsessive exercise fanatics any more than we need a nation of couch potatoes. What we need is a nation of people who realize that regular, moderate exercise can dramatically extend and enrich their lives – and who act accordingly.

How far you run or how much you lift today is relatively unimportant. It's the regular, ongoing exercise you continue to do a year from now, five years from now and 10 years from now that will make the difference in how well you feel, how good you look and how long you live.

Today's New-Look Gyms

When I first developed an interest in bodybuilding, it wasn't easy to find a suitable place to train. Health clubs as we know them today were yet to be invented. Except in the largest cities, public gyms were scarce. Most of them were small, grubby, uninviting places that smelled of liniment and sweat. Their clients were 100 percent male and mostly blue-collar types.

Today, all that's changed. Now you can find a gym on every other corner – almost literally – in most locales, and neither they nor their clientele bears any resemblance to those of 50 years ago. A lot of oldtimers wouldn't know where they were the first time they walked in. For the most part, modern gyms are bright, open, pleasant places, where business and professional men and women go to have a good time as well as to get themselves in shape. They're filled with sophisticated, state-of-the-art exercise equipment for both cardiovascular and weight-resistance exercise. Many of them have jogging tracks for "purists," squash and tennis courts for game-players, and even cocktail lounges for people whose main interest in exercise is bending their elbows.

Seriously, though, I know a lot about gyms. I've run dozens of them myself, and, in fact, I still own a couple. But in recent times, I've leased out my own facilities and become "just another member" at a large, new, well-equipped gym not far from my house. The staff is competent and friendly, the atmosphere is relaxed, and there's every type of machine and free weights I need for a complete workout.

As I mentioned earlier, I don't like to exercise at home, and I don't keep any exercise equipment there. Instead, I spend a couple of hours at the gym at least five days each week. I believe in making exercise as comfortable and convenient as possible, and that's exactly what a good gym does. To me, it's by far the most practical, sensible place to exercise.

Discipline, as I've said before, is the name of the game when it comes to getting fit and staying that way. If you have the discipline to exercise regularly at home, more power to you. But for many of us – myself included – the home environment is simply not conducive to fitness. There are too many distractions, too many comforts, too much food and drink in the refrigerator, and it's too easy to lose focus and concentration.

If you want evidence of how difficult it is to exercise at home, all you have to do is look at the "Sports Equipment" section of the classified ads in your newspaper and see how much unused home exercise gear people are trying to get rid of. For every person who actually rides a stationary bike in the den while watching TV, I suspect you'll find 1,000 home "exercycles" whose only function is to catch dust.

I believe everyone should approach exercise in the way that suits him or her best. My way is to head for the gym.

An Incredible Bargain

Despite their rapidly increasing popularity, millions of Americans still have never set foot inside a gym or health club. If you're one of them, you may have gotten the idea that it costs a lot to be a member. Well, it doesn't. Although prices do vary widely, many memberships represent one of the biggest bargains in today's marketplace -- if you use the facilities the way you should.

Some high-end health clubs charge as much as $120 per month. At the other end of the scale, some charge as little as $12 monthly. But for basic exercise, more expensive doesn't necessarily mean better. The monthly fee at my own gym is just $16, an incredible bargain, considering that this entitles me to as many hours of use as I want during the month. With my normal 10-hour-a-week workout schedule, this comes to less than 40 cents per hour. You can't beat that!

At prices like these, I can't see any justification for the outdoor dangers, discomforts and inconveniences that so many exercisers subject themselves to. Inside a gym, the temperature is always ideal. There's never any rain or snow. No vicious dogs or crazy drivers. No potholes or puppy-poop to step in.

I can't tell you how many times I've seen some poor guy jogging along a sidewalk in 100-degree afternoon heat. I can't think of anything more excruciating than that, and I can't imagine any doctor recommending this kind of exercise. After all, what point is there in protecting yourself against a heart attack only to fall dead of a heat stroke?

If you want to run or jog outdoors and deal with all these hazards and distractions just to save 40 cents an hour, that's your business. But I believe in making exercise comfortable and convenient – and safe – so I'll continue to go to the gym. Let's face it, how many people are going to continue doing something that makes them miserable? The more comfortable we make exercise, the more likely we are to keep doing it – and the more potential benefits it holds for us.

The Social Side of Exercise

There are a number of other advantages to doing your training at a gym in the company of other exercisers. Chances are, you'll find the people working out around you to be considerably friendlier than those you pass as you jog along the sidewalk.

Once you get used to the idea, going to the gym can become an enjoyable social event – more recreation than onerous responsibility. Many gyms offer nurseries for the kids, so that husbands and wives can exercise together.

Exercising with a partner, whether it happens to be your spouse, another relative or just a friend who shares your interest in fitness, can make the routine a lot more pleasant. Having an "exercise buddy" provides moral support as you're getting started, and later gives you someone with whom to compare progress.

Since most modern gyms are coed, they're also an excellent place for a single person to meet members of the opposite sex. Think about it: Would you rather date someone you met in some dark, smoky bar when you were half-crocked or someone who cares enough about his or her health and appearance to go to a gym and exercise?

Unfortunately, many baby boomers in their mid-to-late 40s are now getting divorces and looking for a new "significant other." For them, membership in a health club can serve two important purposes: (1) It can provide a safe, wholesome environment for new social/romantic contacts, and (2) it can help put them in shape to meet the stiff competition in today's "mating game."

As they become comfortable with the atmosphere and surroundings and get to know some of the people they're exercising with, many health club members find themselves spending much more time at the gym than their training program demands. Don't be surprised if you turn out to be one of them.

Follow the Stars' Example

For anyone who can afford it and wants to get super-serious about exercise, the most ideal approach, in my opinion, is to hire a personal trainer to work with you. These highly trained professional fitness instructors can design an individualized fitness program tailored especially for you. Many personal trainers are certified by the American Council on Exercise, and they are genuine experts who can guide you to unprecedented levels of fitness.

More and more top Hollywood stars are using their own personal trainers. I think the trend started when Arnold Schwarzenegger came on the scene with his great physique and made so many other stars look weak and flabby by comparison. Now virtually all the big-name stars have personal trainers – Sylvester Stallone, Barbra Streisand, Oprah Winfrey and Tom Arnold, just to name a few. I understand that Madonna employs no less than three personal trainers who travel with her everywhere she goes.

A personal trainer has the know-how to design a comprehensive training regimen perfectly suited to your needs in the areas of both fitness and appearance. Admittedly, they don't come cheap. The standard fees for personal trainers ranges from $25 to $50 per hour. But if you're financially able, hiring a personal trainer to work with you for a couple of hours a week, even if it's only for a month or two, can pay major dividends.

It's the top-of-the-line approach in the field of fitness. If it's out of your reach, having a partner to motivate and support you is the next best thing.

When you select a personal trainer – if you do – I strongly suggest selecting one who looks the part. Being certified is often of secondary importance. I prefer to be guided by how successful a personal trainer has been in developing his or her own body. If it's the kind of body you've always aspired to have for yourself, chances are you've found the right person for the job.

No "Spot Reducing"

People are always approaching me with questions like: "What kind of exercise should I do to make my stomach smaller?"

To which I sometimes jokingly reply: "Push yourself away from the table three or four times a day."

Actually, there's no such thing as successful "spot reducing." You can tone up the muscles in your thighs or calves or belly by repeating a certain exercise often enough. Or you can slim your whole body by cutting down on calories and fat. Or you can combine the two processes for an even healthier, more attractive result.

But it's not my purpose in this book to go into great detail about specific exercises or to give precise directions on how to do them. There are plenty of other books and pamphlets around with this kind of information. If you buy a piece of exercise equipment, instructions on using it will be included. And if you join a health club or gym, its staff members can usually provide any technical information you may need about how to use the various machines. Do not, however, expect them to serve as instructors. The low fee structure at most gyms simply won't allow for that.

Getting the Most From a Gym

To make sure you get your money's worth from your gym or health club, here are a few things to keep in mind:

(1) If your schedule is flexible enough, set your workouts during the morning or early afternoon. Gym facilities start getting crowded around 5 p.m., when the majority of people get off work, and the crowds tend to build steadily for the next two or three hours. Since I'm not an "early person," I often wait until the period of peak demand has passed and start my workouts around 9 p.m.

(2) It's best to wait for an hour or two after eating to start your workout, but it's also important not to wait too long. You

need to maintain a high blood sugar level to carry you through a period of sustained exercise.

(3) Instead of dosing yourself with coffee, tea or other caffeine-containing drinks to keep you on your toes during exercise, try eating some complex carbohydrates (a couple of whole-wheat crackers, an oatmeal cookie, a rice cake or a few pretzels) to maintain your energy and alertness.

(4) Always remember that a successful exercise program and proper nutrition go hand in hand. It's next to impossible to have one without the other, but that doesn't keep a lot of people from trying. At least nine out of 10 of the men and women I see working out in a gym aren't following a good nutritional program. That's why some of them exercise for years and still end up overweight.

A Look Back at the Basics

Let's take a minute to sum up a few basic points about exercise:

Most important to your good health and long life are cardiovascular or aerobic exercises – walking, jogging, running, cycling, dancing, skipping rope, swimming, etc. Any sport that involves a lot of sustained rapid movement of the whole body, such as tennis, badminton, volleyball, basketball and soccer, also provides some aerobic benefits. But such activities as golf (especially if you ride from hole to hole in a golf cart), bowling, pool, waterskiing, horseshoes and even baseball do very little for the cardiovascular system.

To build and tone muscles, use lifting and other weight-resistance exercises. For suppleness and agility, add bending and stretching exercises. Such old-fashioned calisthenic-style exercises as pushups, situps, kneebends and leglifts still produce the desired results, but today's modern machines do the job better and easier.

Every muscle in your body needs exercise. Something as simple as trying to touch the tip of your tongue to the end of your nose a dozen or so times a day can do wonders to tone up facial muscles and prevent a sagging jawline.

Without exercise, muscles atrophy and fade away. You can see this happening before your very eyes when someone is bedridden for a period of several weeks. The benefits of exercise don't last very long once you stop exercising. Within as little as 21-28 days, fitness and muscle tone can be almost totally lost, and you can regress virtually back to the point of never having exercised at all.

This is why, in order for it to give you a longer, fuller life, exercise should have no "stopping place." It has to become an inseparable, continuous part of you.

Going for days without any vigorous physical exercise and then trying to "do it all" in one big burst of activity is especially dangerous. It can damage your heart and other organs, your joints, your skeletal muscles, your whole body.

But when it's done right – and backed by proper nutrition and supported by a positive attitude – exercise can perform miracles.

That Born-Again Feeling

Not long ago, I went to see a 67-year-old friend with prostate cancer. He looked to have aged 10 years since the last time we'd been together. His mood was bleak. His once-muscular body was frail. He seemed defeated, and I could almost feel him slipping away.

Somehow, I talked him into going to the gym with me. I formulated an exercise program just for him, one that started out slowly and built up gradually because he was in a very weakened condition. I also gave him a low-fat, high-protein, high-carbohydrate nutrition regimen to follow, then worked with him personally for several weeks. I joked with him, complimented him on his progress and motivated him to keep going.

At the end of that time, I was rewarded by seeing a totally changed man. He still has cancer, but he looks better than he has in years. He says he feels much better, too. And his psychological outlook is more positive than that of many people who are supposedly in perfect health.

"I feel like I've been born again," he says.

In a sense, he has been. You can be, too.

"In America, the young are always ready to give to those who are older than themselves the full benefits of their experience."
–OSCAR WILDE

CHAPTER

7

Fiscal Fitness – What the Big Corporations Have Learned

Over the past few years, scores of major U.S. corporations have made an amazing discovery -- one they probably should have made decades ago: Employees who participate in organized programs of exercise, fitness and "wellness" are worth more to their companies in dollars and cents than those who don't.

Obviously, workers who are fit and healthy lose less time to sickness, and this factor alone makes them more valuable. It doesn't take an economics professor to figure that out. But according to studies conducted by several large employers, those who stay fit through exercise are also more productive, more dependable, more amicable toward management and co-workers, less likely to have accidents and less likely to quit or be fired. In addition to stronger, more durable bodies, they have higher morale, greater self-esteem and keener minds. And, as an added bonus, they can sharply reduce their company's health insurance costs by lowering the number of claims.

It adds up to this deceptively simple equation: Physically fit employees equal fiscally fit companies. Employee fitness is an important asset that can make a striking difference in the corporate bottom line.

Exercise is Good Business

Because of this discovery, an increasing number of companies are making major investments in company gyms and fitness centers and even arranging to let employees exercise on company time. This is a nice fringe benefit for employees – but it's also much more. It's another in a growing list of reasons why nobody "doesn't have time" to exercise these days. In addition to company-sponsored programs, more and more community centers, schools, colleges and hospitals are offering free or inexpensive fitness and wellness programs.

Corporate management hasn't gotten so deeply involved in the fitness movement out of the goodness of its heart, of course. Companies have learned it's just good business to encourage their employees to exercise. For every dollar invested in fitness, the companies can expect to get several dollars in return.

In all likelihood, they will double or triple their investment, based on the experience of numerous companies that have pioneered the fitness concept. Blue Cross Blue Shield of Indiana had a 250-percent return on its investment in a corporate fitness program – or $2.51 for every $1 invested over a five-year period – according to the *American Journal of Health Promotion*.

Other companies have reported even more impressive returns. In the first year of its TriHealthalon employee fitness program, General Mills received a payback of $3.10 per $1 invested. In the second year, the payback jumped to $3.90.

Motorola, meanwhile, reported a $3.15 return and PepsiCo a $3 return for each $1 invested. Over a four-year period, Kennecott Copper Company had a return of $5.78. And Coors Brewing Company reported an average annual return of $6.15 during the first six years its fitness program was in operation.

Companies Save Millions

Let's take a look at some other actual examples of how fitness is saving big bucks for corporate America:

In a three-year study, DuPont found it saved $1.6 million during the first year of its fitness program. The second-year savings were about the same, $1.5 million. But in the third year, the savings jumped to $3 million, according to a report in the *American Journal of Public Health*. Absenteeism fell by more than 47 percent among participants in the DuPont program over a six-year period.

General Electric reduced health care costs for members of its fitness program by 38 percent in an 18-month period, while the cost for non-members was rising by 21 percent. Costs for fitness program participants averaged $757 annually in contrast to a yearly cost of $941 for non-participants. GE also found that employees who exercised were absent from work 45 percent fewer days than employees who didn't.

After Mesa Petroleum instituted an employee fitness program, its health care costs per employee rose only 4.8 percent, compared to a national average in the same year of 105 percent. Annual health care costs per employee were $1,121 for Mesa, compared to the national average of $3,560. In addition, says Mesa Chairman T. Boone Pickens: "Our fitness program saves Mesa more than $200,000 in insurance claims annually."

Over a six-year period, medical claims costs were 55 percent lower for employees of Steelcase Corporation who took part in its corporate fitness program than for those who didn't. The average claim for participants was $478.61 versus $869.98 for non-participants.

Getting That Mental Edge

The spin-off benefits of fitness programs seem to go on and on, and not all of them are physical. They give participants a mental and psychological edge, too. For example:

General Motors found that employees in its program had a 50-percent reduction in job grievances, a 50-percent reduction in on-the-job accidents and a 40-percent reduction in lost time.

In a survey of Union Pacific Railroad employees, 75 percent expressed the belief that regular exercise helped them achieve a higher level of concentration and relaxation at work. Eight out of 10 credited their exercise program with helping them be more productive on the job.

The Canadian Life Assurance Company reported that 47 percent of participants in a fitness program were more alert, had better rapport with co-workers and supervisors, and enjoyed their work more than those who didn't participate. Even more,

63 percent, said they were more relaxed, more patient and less tired during the work day.

There's strong evidence that executives who work out regularly are better decision makers. When the decision-making capabilities of 80 people were monitored over a nine-month period, researchers at Purdue University found that exercisers' ability to make complex decisions had improved by 70 percent over non-exercisers.

The Government Joins In

Government agencies are also getting into the act, both at the local and national level.

Participants in an exercise control program at NASA were found to have improved stamina and work performance, as well as enhanced concentration and decision-making abilities. Compared to the average office worker, whose efficiency decreases by 50 percent during the final two hours of the working day, exercisers were able to work at full efficiency all day long, resulting in a 12.5 percent increase in productivity.

On average, police officers are almost certainly more physically fit than the average person, but organized fitness programs also help keep them free of illness. The Dallas Police Department reported that the amount of sick time taken by participants in its fitness program decreased by 29 percent while non-participants were losing 5 percent more days in sick leave.

This is how Dr. D. W. Edington of the University of Michigan sums up the economic impact of organized fitness programs on the companies and agencies that sponsor them:

"Wellness programs in general and fitness programs in particular may be the only employee benefits which pay money back. When more people come to work, you don't need to pay overtime or temporary help; when people stay at the job longer, training costs go down; lower health care claims cost you less if you're self-insured – and health care insurers as well as some companies are already beginning to create premiums based on fitness levels."

Disproving a False Notion

With all the evidence accumulated in recent years, companies no longer have to speculate or suppose what benefits might result from higher levels of employee fitness. Now they know beyond the shadow of a doubt that employees who exercise and take care of themselves mean less waste, higher morale, greater productivity, smoother operations – and most of all, higher profit margins.

The most important contribution of fitness programs, however, isn't the money they save. It isn't even the more pleasant, more productive atmosphere they produce in the workplace. By far their greatest contribution is the better health and longer lives they produce for the people who take part in them.

Like the exercise/nutrition programs conducted by millions of individual Americans, the company programs open up exciting new vistas for those of us in our middle years. They show us that if we take proper care of ourselves, we can do more, feel better, look better and function longer than our grandparents ever imagined possible.

The insurance actuaries haven't yet calculated how much an ongoing, comprehensive fitness program adds to average life expectancy. In the near future, they undoubtedly will, and when they do, companies will have another vital reason to push their programs.

Clearly, the implications of these programs for over-50 employees are vast and far-reaching. With every passing month, more employers are realizing that your state of health and fitness has a lot more to do with your value as an employee than your age. In the process, they are finally getting away from the false notion that advancing age and ill health always go hand in hand.

Generally, this is extremely good news, both for progressive companies and their older employees, especially those who want or need to keep working beyond the "normal" retirement age of 65. If healthy, able-bodied, mentally alert senior employees stay on the job longer, the company gets greater use of their experience, know-how and leadership abilities. Meanwhile, it also saves the cost of training someone younger to take their place.

If you're in good health and you're a good producer for your company, why shouldn't you work as long as you want? The question demands an answer. And the demand will only grow louder as time goes on.

Companies with enlightened management know they have too much at stake economically to continue to turn healthy, productive workers "out to pasture" automatically when they reach a certain birthday. They realize that if a 65-year-old employee is an active participant in a fitness or wellness program, he or she may be worth more to the company than two non-participating 35-year-olds with track records of illness and absenteeism.

Boost Your Earning Power

But as much sense as it makes from the company's standpoint to extend the working life of healthy older workers, the benefits are even greater – and more crucially important – to the individual employee.

Think for a moment what a tremendous difference an additional 10 or 15 years of earned income could mean to you. Because of your advanced skills and long experience, these earnings would likely be at peak levels – possibly two or three times as much as you earned during the early years of your career.

At an annual salary of, say, $40,000, an extra 15 working years would mean an additional $600,000 in earned income. It would mean more time to pay off a home mortgage, reduce overall indebtedness, build savings accounts or IRAs, and make lucrative investments. Instead of relegating yourself to a survival-level existence as a retiree – an existence made more tenuous and insecure by the precarious state of Social Security – these extra years can give you the power to control your own economic destiny.

Considering this, it's no wonder that a recent CNN poll of baby boomers showed the majority of them were approaching their 50th birthdays with plans to work until age 75 or beyond if they had that option. Today's typical wage earners simply want – and usually need – more time to prepare themselves financially for a comfortable, meaningful retirement.

Besides, if we're going to live to 100 or beyond, we can work until we're in our 80s and still have 20 or so years to loll in the sun and smell the roses.

Coming Apart at the Seams

The harsh reality of the situation, though, is that even those who would continue to choose drawing retirement benefits at the traditional age of 65 may not have that opportunity much longer. For anyone under 40, the chances of drawing Social

Security benefits are getting slimmer every day. Most younger workers realize this and are preparing themselves for the worst. As *Time* magazine noted not long ago, more people under age 35 believe in UFOs than believe they'll receive payments from Social Security when they hit retirement age.

Sadly, barring some miracle, they're probably right. But workers in their 30s at least have decades to make adjustments. It's those of us over 50 who are going to feel the pinch first, and we have less time for effective counter-measures.

The most hopeful projections give Social Security about 20 years before calamity strikes – in the form of tens of millions of those same baby boomers reaching what we today consider retirement age. If our system foolishly continues to force or entice most of these people out of the labor force and onto the Social Security rolls at 65, the system will collapse. The only way to salvage it will be through gigantic tax increases or sharp cuts in benefits – or both.

The unravelling of Social Security, however, has already started. Up until 1995, almost all Social Security recipients could expect to get back everything they had contributed during their working years, plus interest, within a few years after retirement. After that, each benefit check represented a profit.

A Losing Proposition

But some 1995 retirees will become the first losers under the system. If you calculate the interest they might have drawn on the money they paid in Social Security taxes, assuming they had put that same amount into a savings account instead, the benefits they draw will fall short of what they've "contributed" during their working years. *Time* calls this a "bad deal." I agree, but I also know it's only the beginning. It's bound to get worse.

To illustrate the shortfall between Social Security benefits and the return that could be expected from wise private investment, *Time* cites this example: If the total Social Security contribution by a wage earner and his employer were $92,000, the wage earner would draw a Social Security benefit of $1,135 per month if he retired at 65. But by investing that same amount in short-term Treasury notes, the retiree could have bought an annuity worth $1,295 per month. Or he could have put his money into corporate bonds that would give him $1,880 per month.

For our purposes here, there's very little point in trying to figure out how our government got Social Security into this mess or how it can get it out. Congress will no doubt be grappling with that question for years to come. A lot of people are to blame for what's happening, but that's beside the point. The point is, we're there – in deep water and far from shore. What the federal bureaucracy will do in its attempts to remedy the situation is anybody's guess. Judging from some of its past bonehead moves, nothing is too stupid, shortsighted or self-defeating for the government to try.

My advice while waiting for a solution is "Don't hold your breath." Time and again, Washington has shown an amazing talent for dodging both responsibility and reality. The only safe assumption is that the responsibility for financial self-preservation after age 65 now falls on the individual citizen. In other words, it's every man for himself.

Three Keys to Job Security

One obvious remedy is to keep working longer and use our extra years of earning capacity to construct our own personal financial safety net without total dependence on Social Security.

But our ability to do this hinges on four main factors: (1) We have to convince our employers that it's worth their while to keep us on the payroll after we turn 65. (2) We have to keep ourselves fit, healthy and alert enough to continue to earn our keep. (3) We have to be able to compete with younger workers for the same jobs. And (4) we have to look the part.

We can probably expect some additional incentives from the beleaguered Social Security Administration for staying on the job. In all likelihood, for example, those who wait until age 70 or 75 to retire will be offered increased monthly benefits when they do quit working. But the cynical underlying hope will be that these older recipients don't live long enough to break even.

Meanwhile, in order to maintain the illusion of "full employment," there will be simultaneous pressure from other portions of the federal government for workers to retire at the usual age, even if there's nothing to retire on. With Social Security disintegrating around us, this seems totally illogical – and it is. Yet in the tradition of a two-headed jackass (or elephant, if you prefer) pulling against itself, this is exactly what we should expect from Washington.

Fierce Competition Ahead

For more than a decade, the nation's economy has been generating fewer and fewer jobs for highly paid skilled workers. The bulk of the jobs being created are in the $5-to-$7 per hour range – servers, deliverymen, clerks, laborers, domestic workers, etc.

This means fierce competition in years to come for a shrinking pool of desirable jobs. In many cases, it will be a matter of youth versus age. We will be pitting our experience and accumulated skills against younger people's willingness to work for lower pay. For those of us in the over-50 age group, our physical condition and the way we act and look may spell the difference between having a job and not having one.

Until the relatively recent past, if you worked for the same company for 25 or 30 years, you could expect to stay there until you retired. But suddenly all that has changed. As hundreds of thousands of people who have been caught in corporate layoffs and "downsizings" now realize, there's really no such thing as long-term job security anymore.

Being thrown out of work is traumatic enough when you're in your 20s or 30s. When you're past 40, it gets even tougher. That's when you first start to experience age discrimination, and with each succeeding year, it grows steadily worse. In some fields, it's next to impossible to find a job if you're much past 50.

So imagine yourself at age 65 or beyond, making the rounds of employment offices and personnel managers, urgently seeking the type of job that can give you the financial security your government is no longer able to provide. Not a comforting picture, right?

Now suppose your chief competition for this job is a guy in his late 30s. What kind of chance do you realistically have of beating him out?

Maybe better than you think, if –

You've kept yourself physically fit through regular exercise and proper nutrition.

You act – and feel – sharp, alert and vigorous.

And you look youthful, in-shape and well groomed.

"Eye of the Tiger"

It's important to remember that in the job market, first impressions are everything. The first 30 seconds of any job interview are crucial. If you make a negative impression during those initial 30 seconds, the chances are you'll never recover. And nothing can register as a greater negative in the mind of a personnel director than someone who looks tired, lethargic, disspirited or unhealthy.

"To overcome age prejudices during a job interview, it's important to stand erect, walk with a bounce in your step and portray vitality, stamina and high self-esteem," says Martin Birnbach, a business analyst for a Dallas radio station. "Older job applicants need to develop that hard-hitting 'eye of the tiger' attitude and mannerism that says, 'I'm ready for anything!' In the employer's mind, these characteristics imply productivity and high performance."

That's almost impossible to do, of course, if you feel weak, demoralized, doubtful of your own capabilites and generally "over the hill." Birnbach points out that people in their 50s, 60s and 70s bring many assets to the employment interview table, including maturity, judgment, patience, a track record of achievement, good work ethic and accrued wisdom. They also are usually free of the stress impacts of raising and educating children and don't usually suffer the radical emotional swings of people in their 20s and 30s.

Yet without that "eye of the tiger" posture and the positive energy to back it up, they still may lose out to someone younger. Employers may question their ability to fit in with or take direction from younger workers.

I've employed hundreds of people in dozens of different capacities during my varied careers, and I can honestly say I'd almost always hire someone over 50 who meets these criteria in preference to a younger person if everything else about them seemed equal.

Experience, maturity and demonstrated dependability carry a lot of weight with me, and I think most employers feel the same. If an older job applicant exudes as much energy, confidence and vitality as a younger candidate, his chronological age wouldn't bother me a bit. If an older guy seems just as bright, imaginative and on his toes mentally as someone 25 years younger, I'd again be swayed in his direction.

I'd also take a long, hard look at each applicant's appearance. This isn't a matter of vanity. It's what our society and the modern workplace demand. A trim person of 65 would get my vote over a 35-year-old who was 50 or 60 pounds overweight. An older person who was neat and well-dressed would rate well ahead of a younger slob. If a younger candidate showed the effects of such destructive habits as smoking, heavy drinking or drug abuse, he would quickly lose ground to an older candidate who didn't.

For the most part, we're talking plain, everyday common sense. In a society where working to age 75 or 80 is destined to become the accepted norm, I have no doubt that most employers will eventually be guided as much by these common-sense factors as by age.

So it's up to each of us in the over-50 age group to stay competitive in the way we look, act, think and feel. If we are to expand our working lives and safeguard our economic future, this will be a necessity.

If you're fortunate enough to work for a company that offers a fitness program, you owe it to yourself to take advantage of it. While it's making you a healthier, happier person, it may also be lowering your health and life insurance premiums. And it can give you some major advantages in the competitive, insecure climate we face tomorrow.

On the other hand, if you don't have access to a corporate program, it's time to act on your own to ensure and protect your personal fitness.

In many ways, it could be an even greater asset than your job itself.

> "Nature abhors the old, and old age seems the only disease; all others run into this one."
> –Ralph Waldo Emerson

CHAPTER

8

Drugs to Slow Aging (and How to Get Around the FDA)

What's your greatest fear? Your worst nightmare? For most people in their middle years, it probably isn't the prospect of dying. By the time we reach our 50s or 60s, we've usually come to terms with our own mortality. We can accept the inevitability of death, although we'd like to postpone it as long as possible. What most of us fear far more than death itself, I think, is the possibility of being left physically or mentally disabled for years -- maybe even decades -- by the ravages of some disease.

Winding up as a helpless "vegetable" – now that's a truly scary thought.

In my opinion, the best way to ensure that this never happens is to start taking preventive measures against the most destructive and widespread diseases that prey on the over-50 population long before the first symptoms appear. We've already discussed some of these measures, such as regular exercise and proper nutrition. But other preventatives come in the form of pills and capsules – medicines that protect healthy people by counteracting their tendencies toward certain illnesses.

I call them "wonder drugs." I take a half-dozen or more varieties of them every day in the firm belief that they'll help me fight off disease and maintain my physical and mental capabilities until I'm 100 or more. I believe just as firmly that they can do the same for you.

This is no pipe dream, friends. There's no hocus-pocus involved here. These drugs are clinically tested, down-to-earth realities. As little-known as most of them are in this country, they're available today – right now. And many scientific studies over the years show they have remarkable abilities to extend life by shielding us from the most dreaded age-related illnesses of the mind and body known to mankind.

I'm talking about Parkinson's Disease, Alzheimer's Disease, diabetes, arthritis, depression, heart disease, stroke, even cancer. Research shows that today's wonder drugs can give an extra measure of protection against all these killers and disablers. They can also bolster and strengthen the all-important immune system against the inroads of advancing age – damage that can lead to the breakdown of the body's defenses against all kinds of lethal invaders.

Prevention Not Allowed

In Europe, Mexico and other parts of the world, these drugs are readily available to anyone. Yet at least 95 percent of Americans don't even know they exist. Only a handful of American physicians are aware of their potential benefits. And unfortunately, if the FDA has its way, the U.S. public and medical profession may not have reliable information about these drugs in our lifetimes, much less ready access to them.

Why? Why would an agency of our own government block our ability to obtain drugs to prevent the world's most destructive disease processes? The answer is paradoxical. They want to "protect" us from "unapproved" substances. But some of these wonder drugs have been tested and researched for decades, and their value is widely recognized in other countries. It looks to me as if the FDA's chief interest is in protecting its own power, not in protecting the public.

Under current law, the FDA can approve drugs only for existing disease conditions. This means that drug therapy aimed at preventing disease in healthy people can't be sanctioned. Therefore, U.S. pharmaceutical companies have absolutely zero initiative to develop preventive drugs, since they couldn't market them if they did. Furthermore, aging is not considered a disease by FDA definitions, so any drug regimen to prevent the debilitating effects of aging is doubly damned.

As part of its ongoing campaign to restrict health freedom in this country, the FDA has sought – unsuccessfully so far – to have vitamin supplements classified as drugs and to make them available only by prescription. The FDA also attacks so-called "alternative medicine" at every opportunity and sometimes tries to harass and intimidate people who buy "unapproved" drugs from sources in other countries.

But all Americans should know that, because of a little-known 1988 change by the FDA in its own regulatory policies, each of us now has the right to obtain supplies of these drugs for our own personal use. The change resulted primarily from pressure by AIDS support groups who charged that AIDS victims were being denied access to potentially life-saving substances that were widely used in other countries.

Legal But Hard to Find

Because of this change, wonder drugs that are available abroad but not approved for sale in the United States may now be lawfully mail-ordered in small quantities by U.S. purchasers so long as they aren't intended for redistribution or resale.

There are, of course, no guarantees that the FDA won't abruptly change its mind and reverse its mail importation policy. And it strictly prohibits any advertising that would help consumers locate sources for unapproved drugs. In the meantime, though, the relaxed rule means a major breakthrough in potential disease prevention and an opportunity for a longer, fuller life for all of us. Until recently, wonder drugs were totally beyond the reach of most U.S. citizens. Now all that has changed.

The drugs aren't always easy to find, though, even today. Don't bother asking your doctor about most of them, for instance. Chances are, he's never heard of them. Not only are 99 out of every 100 U.S. physicians unfamiliar with the drugs, but the risk of malpractice suits would be far too high for most

Drugs To Slow Aging

of them to prescribe unapproved medications, anyway. But now, at last, there are ways to get them.

I recently ordered a supply of several key wonder drugs from a source in the Czech Republic. I've also found many of them in Mexico. I'll tell you more a little later about how to get the drugs themselves and how to obtain reliable information on the ones that may be most appropriate for you.

At this point, you may be telling yourself, "Wow, these things are probably so expensive I couldn't afford them, anyway!" If so, get ready for a pleasant surprise. In comparison with many of the prescription drugs routinely sold in this country, the wonder drugs are very reasonably priced. You can take the recommended daily dosage of three or four of the most important ones for as little as $10 or $12 a week. Almost anyone can afford to spend that much for such tremendous potential benefits.

Protecting the Prostate

My personal interest in preventive and life-extending drugs has grown steadily over the years. One of my first major ventures into this area came after I read about the high incidence of prostate enlargement and prostate cancer among over-50 men. Almost half the U.S. male population suffers benign prostate hypertrophy (BPH), which causes inflammation and painful and frequent urination. One of every seven men in this age group will be diagnosed with prostate cancer during his lifetime.

About the same time, I also learned about a natural herbal compound called saw palmetto that had been been used successfully in Europe for more than a decade to shrink benign enlarged prostate glands.

When a routine medical exam showed my own prostate to be slightly enlarged, I asked my urologist about saw palmetto, and I was somewhat surprised – although I guess I shouldn't have been – when he told me he had never heard of it. Instead, he recommended a new drug called Proscar, which had recently been approved by the FDA.

Since I don't believe in taking anything until I know about its potential side effects, I also did some research on Proscar. What I discovered was that, not only is it expensive (about $60 per month), it can also cause severe side effects, including sexual

_d my doctor, "Thanks, but no thanks. I want to
_e."

_g four capsules (320 milligrams) daily of saw
_e. It costs approximately one-fifth as much as
_ and it has no discernible side effects. Unlike most wonder drugs, it's also easy to obtain, which is an added plus. As an herbal extract not classified as a medication, it's available as an over-the-counter item in many health food stores.

According to the Life Extension Foundation, the saw palmetto herb is a "multisite" inhibitor of the hormone DHT, which plays a major role in the development of prostate disorders. Saw palmetto inhibits 50 percent of the binding of DHT to receptor sites in the prostate. It also blocks uptake of DHT by prostate cells.

Saw palmetto achieved dramatic success in a controlled clinical trial involving 94 patients with enlarged prostates. The 50 who were treated with saw palmetto urinated less frequently, had better urine flow and less pain and discomfort than those who received a placebo. And there were actually fewer adverse side effects in the patients receiving saw palmetto than in the 44 control patients. Not a single man receiving saw palmetto reported any symptoms of impotency.

Recently, saw palmetto has been combined with Pygeum, an extract of the bark of an ancient African tree, to produce even better results than saw palmetto alone in reducing prostate inflammation.

Preventing Mental Decline

Remember that "worst nightmare" I mentioned at the beginning of this chapter? To me, diseases that disrupt and destroy mental function are somehow even more frightening than those that attack the physical body. My father died of Parkinson's Disease, which does both, and being a realist, I feel I may have inherited a genetic tendency to contract Parkinson's at some point in life myself. (Actually, some scientists believe that anyone who lives long enough will eventually develop Parkinson's – and I intend to live a long time.)

Like so many other people in their mid-years, I'm also concerned about Alzheimer's. I can't imagine anything more horrifying than discovering, as former President Ronald Reagan recently did, that you're losing your mind to an irreversible disease process. What could be more demoralizing than knowing you will soon be totally and pathetically dependent on your loved ones to care for your every need as long as you live?

At any rate, much of my interest in wonder drugs has been focused on those with demonstrated abilities in the area of cognitive enhancement. Even if there's no history of Alzheimer's or Parkinson's in your family and you feel your chances of contracting these diseases are remote, almost everyone expects some loss of memory and mental sharpness as the years go by.

Now there's strong scientific evidence that certain chemical compounds – or "Smart Drugs," as they're called in two recent books on the subject – not only preserve and enhance our natural cognitive abilities but also prevent the development of Alzheimer's and Parkinson's. These drugs are vital in combatting such newly defined and extremely common disorders as age-related mental decline (ARMD) and age-associated mental impairment (AAMI), which affect countless Americans.

The "Anti-Aging Drug"

One of the most important of these drugs is deprenyl, which was developed some 40 years ago by Hungarian scientist Jozsef Knoll and has been the subject of intensive research since the 1950s.

Deprenyl has been used to treat Parkinson's Disease in millions of patients, but only recently has it been recognized for its powerful anti-aging qualities. Its amazing ability to extend the lifespan of laboratory animals has won it praise as "today's most promising therapy in the struggle against aging" and the nickname "the anti-aging drug." It is marketed in the U.S. under the trade name Eldepryl.

The results of laboratory tests and clinical trials involving deprenyl are nothing short of phenomenal. The maximum lifespan of rats given deprenyl increased by 40 percent – the equivalent of a human being living to the age of 150! At the same time, the test animals' average lifespan also increased as the aging process slowed. If the animal research holds true for humans, a 100-year-old man or woman taking sufficient doses of deprenyl could be expected to look and feel like a person of 60.

Results of several studies also show that deprenyl can be a potent new weapon against Alzheimer's. Patients treated daily with deprenyl had significant improvements in memory, attention, language abilities and information processing.

Deprenyl is known to increase the sex drive in male laboratory animals, and many men who take it regularly also report increased libido. This is an important extra benefit that probably relates to the general slowing-down of the aging process, since a loss of sex drive is a major symptom of aging. Clincial studies in Europe also show deprenyl to be highly effective in relieving depression. More than 90 percent of depressed patients taking the drug in an Austrian study experienced either full remission or moderate improvement in their condition.

Of Chocolate and Lovers

Chemically, deprenyl is related to phenylethylamine, a substance found in chocolate which also occurs in above-normal quantities in the brains of males and females when they "fall in love." It works in the brain by increasing the levels of dopamine, a neurotransmitter which is crucial to sex drive, motor control, immune function and motivation. The drop in the amount of dopamine-containing neurons in the brain after age 45 is a key factor in the aging process.

Deprenyl is extremely safe, has few undesirable side effects and a low level of toxicity. Some researchers are predicting that it will one day be recognized as a general preventive treatment for age-related degenerative diseases affecting the brain. Much more research is needed, of course. But in the meantime, I think anyone who wants to slow down the aging process and protect himself or herself against Parkinson's and Alzheimer's should be taking deprenyl regularly.

For healthy people 45 and older, a gradually increasing daily dosage is recommended, beginning with 2 or 3 milligrams daily at age 45 or 50 and climbing in increments to 10 milligrams a day at age 80. The recommended dosage for people with diagnosed Parkinsonism is 5 to 10 milligrams daily. Taking too much deprenyl or increasing the dosage too rapidly can cause symptoms of overstimulation, including nausea, irritability, insomnia and nightmares.

As Eldepryl, deprenyl is available all over the U.S. and Canada with a doctor's prescription, although many physicians are reluctant to prescribe it unless a patient already has Parkinson's. It can also be obtained without prescription by mail-order from various overseas suppliers.

An Amazing Hormone

In the next few pages, I want to tell you about several of the other wonder drugs I take every day and let you judge for yourself whether they can be beneficial to you. Some, like deprenyl, are life-extending and cognitive-enhancement drugs. Some are primarily for strengthening the immune system. Still others are aimed at more specific problems affecting health and well-being.

DHEA is a hormone produced by the adrenal glands that has wide-ranging effects on health and longevity. Some scientists believe the level of DHEA in a person's blood can predict his or her future chances of developing such degenerative diseases as diabetes, cancer and atherosclerosis. Memory disorders, learning ability and possibly even aging itself may be affected by these levels.

As you grow older, DHEA levels fall steadily. At 80, you produce only 10 to 20 percent as much DHEA as you produced before your 20th birthday. High blood levels of DHEA are associated with a lower incidence of heart attacks, strokes, malignant tumors and the loss of insulin sensitivity that leads to diabetes. DHEA also protects against bacterial and viral infections and enhances the immune system.

This hormone is remarkably safe – even safer, in fact, than such over-the-counter products as Tylenol, Sudafed, Motrin or even aspirin, according to *Health & Healing* magazine. In terms of any physical risk, it is far safer than most other prescription drugs.

When a person takes regular doses of DHEA, the body tends to utilize it if it needs it and ignore it if it doesn't. If the hormone is given to an animal with a viral infection, for example, the animal will use all the DHEA to enhance its immune system. But if the animal is free of infection or disease, the DHEA is not absorbed by its body. This indicates that there is little or no chance of overdosing on DHEA.

A number of forward-thinking physicians are now prescribing DHEA for patients with diabetes or pre-diabetic symptoms, as well as other degenerative disease processes. Unlike such patented and widely prescribed diabetes drugs as DiaBeta and Micronase, DHEA doesn't increase the risk of cardiovascular disease.

One of the most striking effects of DHEA is its ability to cause weight loss. Studies at Temple University in the 1980s showed that, even when laboratory animals receiving the hormone eat as much as they want, they don't gain weight. Other animals that were obese as a result of high-calorie diets lost weight quickly when they were given DHEA.

Although DHEA is completely legal, it remains an "experimental" drug as far as the FDA is concerned, and the tyrannical government bureaucrats persist in over-controlling it and even trying to penalize doctors who prescribe it. Because it's a cheap, unpatentable therapy, the big pharmaceutical companies would lose tons of money if it should replace their costly – and largely ineffective – drugs for diabetes.

Well, I say to hell with the FDA. The many positive effects of DHEA in preventing diabetes and many other degenerative diseases, as documented by various studies, make it a must on my list of wonder drugs. The optimal dose hasn't yet been established, but I take two 250-milligram tablets daily, which falls somewhere in the mid-range of commonly used dosages. My DHEA was non-existent when I was first tested. Now it's at the level of a person in his early 20s.

In my view, there's no logical reason why anyone shouldn't replace the DHEA lost by the human body as it ages. It's really the only prudent thing to do.

"Medicine" for Healthy People

Piracetam is among the most-studied and best-known of the family of "nootropic" (a Greek term for substances that enhance the mind) or intelligence-boosting drugs. But unlike other drugs of this type, piracetam also effectively enhances many different aspects of human performance. This is why it has become perhaps the most popular wonder drug among normal, healthy people.

One of the scores of studies conducted on piracetam showed that it improves both physical and mental performance in low-oxygen environments, such as high altitudes. Skiers on high mountain slopes, for example, would not only enjoy their sport more, but would also be less likely to injure themselves if they took piracetam. Other studies show that piracetam may protect cigarette smokers from disease processes related to low levels of oxygen in the blood, such as emphysema and atherosclerosis.

But the most intriguing quality of piracetam is its ability to improve cognitive ability in normal people unaffected by any disease process. In a Swedish test, a group of healthy men and women aged 50 and over with above-average IQs were given various performance tests before and after taking piracetam. All showed improvement in every category after receiving the drug.

Piracetam also has great potential for counteracting the type of senility that isn't caused by loss of blood flow due to vascular disease. A study of 84 geriatric patients suffering from this condition showed piracetam improved memory, attention span and general behavior. Piracetam has also improved the cognitive abilities of epileptic patients without interfering with their anti-seizure medications.

Piracetam comes in capsules or tablets of 400 or 800 milligrams, and the usual dose is 2,400 to 4,800 milligrams daily. I take one of the 800-milligram tablets three times a day, which puts me at the low end of the recommended dosage.

Like so many wonder drugs, piracetam remains on the FDA's "black list." Despite decades of totally safe use and millions of prescription and over-the-counter sales in dozens of countries, it's still unavailable in the U.S., but it can be mail-ordered from a number of foreign suppliers. I recently obtained a supply from a European company, then found a short time later that I could buy the drug over the counter in Mexico at about half the European price.

"Smart Pills" Vs. Senility

Some authorities consider hydergine the most important "smart pill" available in the U.S. today. While enhancing mental capabilities, it acts in a variety of ways to slow down or even reverse certain aging processes in the brain.

Among its more significant effects are increasing blood supply and oxygen to the brain. It also protects the brain from damage when the oxygen supply is temporarily insufficient and prevents the damage that oxygen free radicals can cause to brain cells. One of its first uses in the 1940s was as a blood-pressure-lowering drug. It has also lowered abnormally high cholesterol levels in some cases. And it has the ability to increase intelligence, memory, learning and recall.

Hydergine is derived from ergo, a fungus that grows on rye. It has proved to be one of the most effective senility-fighting drugs yet developed. One of the principal causes of senility is hardening of the arteries that supply blood and oxygen to the brain, and no less than 22 authoritative studies have demonstrated hydergine's effectiveness in improving the brain function of senile patients.

Even the FDA recognizes hydergine's tremendous value in treating senile dementia and related circulatory problems, and the drug is approved for those uses. But it's also been shown that patients who receive the drug in higher dosages – 4.5 to 6 milligrams daily – show the greatest improvement. In Europe, dosages of up to 9 milligrams per day are approved, but the FDA has refused to approve a daily dosage of more than 3 milligrams.

This means that many patients aren't getting as much benefit as they could from hydergine. And since the only FDA-approved use of the drug is for diagnosed cases of senile dementia or cerebrovascular insufficiency (lack of blood circulation to the brain), hydergine is being completely denied to millions of people with mild or moderate mental deterioration. Highly reliable research shows that these people could be helped by hydergine – that, in fact, the greatest benefit could be for those whose symptoms are less severe – but Big Brother says no.

Because it definitely can slow or reverse important symptoms of aging, I recently added 5 milligrams daily of hydergine to my personal wonder drugs regimen. It has no serious side effects and is available by prescription anywhere in the country.

Versatile "Youth Drug"

KH3 is an oral form of the world-famous "youth drug" procaine, which was first produced more than 90 years ago and was one of the world's most widely used – and safest – anesthetics for nearly half a century. In KH3, procaine is combined with another substance called hematoporphyrin, which bolsters its effectiveness.

It wasn't until more than 40 years after its discovery that scientists started discovering procaine's amazingly versatile anti-aging qualities. Beginning in the mid-1950s, studies in clinics and hospitals showed that injections of procaine given over extended periods were potent weapons against many symptoms of aging. A more convenient oral form was later developed, and can now be purchased as KH3 in more than 70 countries.

The U.S., unfortunately, isn't one of them. Even after four decades of medical research, the FDA is still withholding its approval of KH3. But it's available over the counter in Nevada.

In clinical trials, KH3 has improved alertness, concentration and recall skills. At the same time, it has the ability to increase physical strength and stamina and improve athletic performance. It does so by improving circulation in both the brain and the body. It has also proved effective in restoring hearing loss, lowering blood pressure, improving mood and attitude, and reducing stress.

In my judgment, any drug that can produce all these beneficial effects is worth taking, even if you have to order it from overseas. I take one 50-milligram KH3 tablet every day.

A Much-Needed Nutrient

Choline is an essential nutritional element sold over the counter in several forms in most health food stores and many drugstores. The nutrient lecithin contains a valuable type of choline called phosphatidyl choline, or PC, which is important to every cell in the body.

Nerve and brain cells in particular need large amounts of PC to maintain and repair themselves. PC also helps the body metabolize fats and plays a role in regulating blood pressure. Deficiencies of choline can cause massive, rapid damage to the kidneys.

Choline is related to acetylcholine, a neurotransmitter in the brain that plays a key role in memory. In a variety of intelligence and memory tests, Choline has improved the performance of normal, healthy people.

I take 1,000 milligrams of choline daily to make sure I get an adequate supply. Persons suffering from manic depression are advised not to take choline because it can deepen the depressive phase of their illness. It also can cause diarrhea in some people, but has no other noticeable adverse side effects.

Sleep Better, Live Longer

I got excited when I first heard about melatonin, and if you're not familiar with this remarkable drug, I think its exceptional capabilities will excite you, too. Some people call it "the anti-cancer hormone."

Every few weeks, it seems, another scientific article reports more about melatonin's amazing ability to prevent and treat diseases ranging from cancer to Alzheimer's, improve sleep patterns, slow aging, combat stress and depression, and even relieve jet lag.

The miraculous qualities of this natural substance were the subject of a major article in *Newsweek* in July 1995 and of a recently published book entitled The *Melatonin Miracle: Nature's Sex-Enhancing, Disease Fighting, Age-Reversing Hormone* by Dr. William Regelson and Dr. Walter Pierpaoli.

Because melatonin slows down secretion of a hormone necessary for ovulation, scientists are experimenting with it as an ingredient in birth control pills. It also shows strong antioxidant qualities as a scavenger of those free radicals that contribute so much to aging and age-associated diseases. It is also so safe that "You can't kill an animal with melatonin," says Dr. Regelson, a professor of medicine at the Medical College of Virginia. He says, however, that children and pregnant or lactating women shouldn't take it at present.

Incredible as it seems, some scientists now speculate that the major cause of breast cancer in women is a deficiency in melatonin. Women with low levels of melatonin are at high risk for breast cancer, studies show. This has led some health authorities to recommend that every woman over 30 take a melatonin capsule daily at bedtime.

I first got interested in melatonin as a sleep aid. Ever since my days as a professional wrestler, I've been troubled periodically by insomnia, and I was told that melatonin would help me get the natural sleep I need. Melatonin is a hormone secreted by the pineal gland in the brain, which functions as a sort of "biological clock." Its secretion is suppressed during the daytime and stimulated by darkness. You can increase the amount of melatonin your body manufactures by seeing that you get some sunshine regularly and do most of your sleeping when it's dark. But melatonin levels decline sharply with age, often leading to age-related insomnia.

There's no question that melatonin helps me sleep. While the usual dose is about 3 milligrams, I take from 10 to 20 milligrams before I go to bed because my needs are apparently greater than average. It's easy to know if you're taking too much melatonin, because you'll have a tendency to wake up groggy. It's also wise not to stay in bright light after taking it, since that will diminish its effectiveness.

I'm confident that melatonin is helping me in many other

ways, too. One of the nicest things about it is that it's a non-prescription substance that can usually be found or ordered wherever nutritional substances are sold – at least for now. What the FDA might try to do to restrict it in the future is anybody's guess.

Rejuvenating Your Immunity

One of the emerging wonder drugs that I want to know more about and may start taking myself is thymosin, a hormone that may hold some vital keys to both the aging process and the breakdown in immunity that allows cancer to gain a foothold in the body.

Thymosin is produced by the thymus gland, a small organ located below the breastbone that is sort of a control center for the immune system. The thymus gland "instructs" defensive cells in the bone marrow, lymph nodes and spleen to attack any foreign tissue or organism that invades the body.

But about the time of puberty, the thymus gland starts to shrink, and as we grow older, the number of thymosin-producing cells steadily decreases, along with the amount of thymosin in the bloodstream. Thymosin levels are much lower in the elderly than in younger people. The lack of thymosin may weaken the immune system and make us more susceptible to disease. All available evidence suggests that maintaining pre-adolescent levels of thymosin could rejuvenate the immune systems of older people, giving them added years of vigorous good health. But it also indicates that the best time to start giving thymosin is early in life.

Thymosin has been successfully used to improve immune function in children born without functioning thymus glands and as an anti-cancer treatment in conjunction with chemotherapy. The National Cancer Institute conducted one study in which patients with advanced and inoperable lung cancer who received thymosin lived twice as long as those who didn't.

Thymosin was discovered about 30 years ago by Dr. Allan Goldstein, now chairman of the Department of Biochemistry at George Washington University Medical Center in Washington, D.C. Three types of thymosin products are being developed, but the FDA has refused thus far to approve any of them, and the drug is available only on an experimental basis at a few medical centers.

However, it's already on the market in Italy, Germany and

Argentina, and may be available through some overseas sources.

hGH – Boon or Curse?

Unquestionably the world's most controversial drug at the moment is human growth hormone, or hGH, which has been injected into people experimentally since the late 1950s, and the use of which is more hotly debated today than ever before.

This mysterious hormone is produced naturally during sleep by the pituitary gland, a small oval-shaped organ at the base of the brain, and is a powerful force in regulating human growth. Its first medical use was as a highly effective treatment for dwarfism in small children, but later, it was also tested on elderly men in failing health with stunning results – a sharp drop in body fat, a sharp rise in muscle mass and an apparent slowdown in the aging process.

Since a report on these experiments was published in 1990 in the *New England Journal of Medicine*, "longevity clinics" administering hGH have sprung up all over the U.S. and Mexico.

More and more baby boomers are intrigued by the possibility, and more and more parents are pressuring pediatricians to give the hGH to their normal-size children in order to make them bigger and stronger.

Meanwhile, the hormone's ability to stimulate muscle growth, toughen skin and increase bone density has also caught the attention of countless professional athletes. In the same way that competitive-minded athletes experimented with steroids at the risk of serious mental and physical damage, many now see hGH as a "magic bullet" to give them an edge on the playing field or in the arena.

The first hGH came from cadavers, but some of the dead "donors" were found to be contaminated with an agent that caused a potentially deadly brain disease in the recipients. This danger prompted the first serious doubts about the hormone's use, but the problem was apparently eliminated in 1985, when the first synthetic hGH was developed.

Proponents of hGH say it has tremendous promise as a veritable fountain of youth and in some cases has turned back the body's "aging clock" by 20 years or more. Its detractors condemn it as an incredibly dangerous substance that can trigger a Pandora's box of ugly side effects, including arthritis, osteoporosis, hypertension, polyps on the colon, enlarged heart or other organ overgrowth, pituitary tumors and diabetes. Depression, anxiety and other mental disorders have also been blamed on hGH. It was allegedly one of many unauthorized drugs being taken by ex-pro football star Lyle Alzado when he died of brain cancer.

The only approved use of hGH continues to be as a treatment for dwarfism, and the only two "official" U.S. manufacturers have placed strict controls on it. But there is plenty of "counterfeit" human growth hormone available for other uses – if you want to pay the going rate of $1,000 a month for it. At this price, it's well out of the financial reach of most people, but some athletes and other experimenters do have the money to spend and are willing to take the risk.

The possibilities of hGH are fascinating. If you can afford the cost and can take it under a doctor's supervision, it could certainly be worth checking out.

Fortresses Against Disease

There are many other wonder drugs out there that are worth learning more about. Isoprinosine, biostim and hyperforat are powerful immune-system boosters, which have proved effective in preventing viral infections and keeping HIV-positive patients from developing active AIDS. Acetyl L-carnitine or ALC is a powerful compound that benefits the heart, lungs, liver and central nervous system while combatting Alzheimer's Disease and slowing aging. Vasopressin restores loss of memory, improves learning ability and helps cure amnesia.

And so on.

Obviously, it would be impossible – or at least impractical – for any individual to take every wonder drug that might offer potential life-extending, health-protecting and disease-preventing benefits. In all likelihood, few people would even want to take as many of these drugs as I take each day. But I've considered myself a "walking laboratory" for a long time, and I'm eager to gauge the beneficial effects of these substances on my own mind and body.

I think anyone over 50 would be doing himself or herself a favor by taking the recommended dosages of at least one or two immunity-boosting drugs and one or two cognitive-enhancement drugs. But that decision, of course, rests with you.

The idea is to protect ourselves against as many of the principal age-associated disease processes as possible. For the most part, we can guard against heart attacks, strokes and atherosclerosis with proper nutrition and regular exercise. But additional measures are needed to protect us from cancer, degenerative mental disorders and life-threatening infectious diseases.

In short, wonder drugs can help make our bodies the total fortresses against disease that they must become if we are to reach 100. They give us another entire arsenal of defensive weapons in our fight against disease and aging.

If you're not certain about which drugs are right for you, I strongly recommend joining the Life Extension Foundation, a non-profit organization dedicated to freedom of choice in health care. The membership fee is only $75 a year, and I can't think of a better investment in health and longevity. The experts at the Life Extension Foundation can provide valuable information on how to obtain the wonder drugs you need. You can call the foundation toll-free at 1 (800) 841-5433. The mailing address is: P.O. Box 229120, Hollywood, Florida 33022-9120.

If you want more details on any of these drugs, I suggest reading *Smart Drugs & Nutrients* or *Smart Drugs II, The Next Generation* – or both. These two books by Ward Dean, M.D., and John Morgenthaler are among the best published guides to these remarkable substances. Both are available in most bookstores. *The Physician's Guide to Life Extension Drugs*, published by the Life Extension Foundation, is another excellent reference.

Looking Toward Tomorrow

For those who plan to take a variety of wonder drugs, the sources above can be particularly valuable. While none of the drugs has been shown to be toxic, there's always a small risk that certain combinations of substances or overly large doses could produce undesirable side effects. As already mentioned, there's little point in asking your doctor about many wonder drugs, but I encourage you to seek his opinion on those drugs that can be purchased by prescription in the U.S.

Thirty or 40 years from now, many of the drugs I've discussed in this chapter may be taken routinely every day by tens of millions of Americans as standard preventive measures against disease and deterioration. We can hope that, by then, the tyranny of the FDA will have been overturned, and ordinary citizens will have the health freedom they deserve.

But those of us over 50 can't afford to wait until then to start taking these drugs – not if we want to be around to see these marvelous events happen. The time to begin protecting ourselves is right now.

"The art of medicine consists of amusing the patient while nature cures the disease."
—VOLTAIRE

CHAPTER 9

What Your Doctor Won't Tell You (Unless You Ask)

We Americans have a nasty habit of putting our physicians in a no-win situation. We expect and demand too much of them – more than anyone could be expected to deliver – and refuse to carry our fair share of the burden of protecting our own health. Far too many of us have the misguided idea that we can simply turn over all our medical problems and health concerns to the doctor and that our responsibility ends there.

"Fix me, Doc," we say. "Give me a pill to cure what ails me. Give me a pill to make me feel better. Hurry and take care of my problem so I can go right back and start doing the same things that made me sick in the first place."

That sounds stupid, doesn't it? Sure it does. It is stupid. But people do it all the time. How many people do you know who've had a heart attack or a bypass operation, then started smoking again? Or gone right on living on pizza, ice cream, fried chicken and hot dogs? Or refused to exercise or control their weight? Then, three or four years later, when their arteries clog up again and they need another bypass, they blame the doctor – if they're able.

It's no coincidence that a third of the people who survive a first heart attack die within five years of another attack or some related cause. As soon as the initial crisis is past, they revert to the same old deadly habits that caused it in the first place.

Just "Take Your Medicine"

Untold millions of us have conditioned ourselves to believe that a bottle of pills can cure anything. We don't have to give up cigarettes or quit eating cheeseburgers or stop being couch potatoes. All we have to do is "take our medicine like the doctor says" and everything will be just fine.

If you believe that, there's a certain bridge across the East River in New York City that I'd like to sell you – cheap!

There's much more to combatting complex disease processes than popping pills.

As I've emphasized before, a modern physician's focus is usually on a specific health problem in which he rates as a specialist and expert. His aim is to relieve the symptoms of that particular problem. If, in doing so, the treatment creates other problems elsewhere in the human machine, it's up to the patient to have enough intelligence, awareness and self-concern to find out about it and then decide if "curing" one problem justifies the creation of another.

I'm frequently amazed at how many people never bother to ask if there are alternative therapies or medications to what their doctor recommends. They never seek information about the liabilities that may be attached to a certain medication or what else might be available – and so they never know.

Many patients simply don't want to think about their ailments. Whenever a new problem crops up, they prefer swallowing another $4-apiece pill to doing something about the underlying cause. And learning about the possible undesirable side effects is just too much trouble. Millions of people willingly become "prescription junkies" instead of exploring other ways to improve their health. Then, when something goes wrong, they blame the doctor.

Some Upsetting Side Effects

A number of years ago, at a time when I was running a high-stress business with more than 100 employees and real estate investments in the $100 million range, my blood pressure started acting up. During a routine physical exam, my doctor checked it and told me it was pretty high. Not to the dangerous stage at that point, but high enough to be a concern.

"You probably need to be taking something," he said. "I'll give you a prescription."

I took the prescription, had it filled, started taking the medication as directed and didn't think very much more about it for a while. But then I noticed some things that bothered me. I found myself feeling rather lethargic sometimes. Training got noticeably harder. I also noticed that I seemed to be going to the bathroom more often. Within a few weeks, I discovered to my horror that I'd lost at least 15 pounds of solid muscle.

I was pretty sure by now that what I'd been taking was a "water pill" – a diuretic. Since muscles are 70 percent water, this type of medication can have a devastating effect, especially on a bodybuilder.

And worst of all, I realized that my sex drive had dwindled sharply since I began taking the blood pressure medicine. My libido had disappeared almost overnight.

This really worried me. As I've repeatedly stressed in this book – and as I'll discuss in detail in a later chapter – I believe sex is a vital part of life at any age. I certainly intend to remain sexually active as long as I live. I happen to like sex. But more than that, I also believe it to be one of the most significant keys to counteracting the aging process. As long as you enjoy and value sex and consider your own sexuality and sexual performance important, it's easier to remain physically and psychologically youthful.

Learning the Awful Truth

Anyway, I wasn't about to give up my sex life in exchange for lowering my blood pressure a few points – not if I could help it. It was obviously time to start asking my doctor some pointed questions, so I called and made the earliest possible appointment.

"Is this a diuretic you're giving me for my blood pressure?" I asked.

"Yes," he said, "the medication does contain a mild diuretic. Why?"

I told him point-blank what was happening. Then I asked: "Is a loss of libido one of the side effects this medicine can have?"

He nodded. "It's been known to affect some people that way."

"Well, that settles it," I told him. "I'm going to quit taking it as of now and try some other tactics to get my blood pressure down and keep it down."

"Sure, that's fine, Ray," the doctor said. "It's entirely up to you. You might try cutting down on the stress in your life and not eating so much salt. It may take a little more effort and dedication, but you might get just as good results."

Fortunately, my doctor didn't share the attitude that many physicians seem to have about sex and aging. There's a predominant feeling – not just among the medical profession but among the general public, too – that if you're over 50 or so, who cares? The idea is that sex should no longer matter, either because you've somehow outgrown your need for physical intimacy or you simply "can't cut the mustard" anymore.

So what difference does it make if some old geezer takes a pill that makes him impotent? In my book, it makes a helluva lot of difference, but this is part of the age-related "typecasting" that goes on all the time. I've known of old geezers in their 70s who fathered children, and I know plenty of people in their 70s who maintain an active sex life.

A Pill-less Solution

I'll tell you exactly how I solved my problem. I sat down and asked myself a question: "Exactly what is it that's bugging me and keeping me on edge?" I figured out that 85 percent of the people who worked for me were fine employees. But the other 15 percent were grating on my nerves and driving my blood pressure up by being unreliable and/or hard to get along with. So I fired those people, and immediately got rid of my irritation. It was that simple.

I also quit using salt – period. I used to be very free with the salt shaker, and everything tasted a little flat for a while without it, but I was actually amazed at how quickly I lost any craving for salt and how little I missed it. Within a few months, my taste adjusted so completely that I could hardly stand the thought of eating a salty pickle or pretzel. Although I occasionally eat processed food or restaurant food that does contain some salt, I never add salt to food prepared from scratch (as is 95 percent of what I eat), either during the cooking phase or at the table. Consequently, my overall sodium consumption is very low.

Oh yes, my blood pressure is perfectly normal. It averages about 130/80. And I've never once regretted questioning my doctor about those "water pills."

My solution might not work for everybody, but it did work for me. But if I had gone on blindly and unquestioningly taking the pills, I never would have known, and I would have suffered consequences that were totally unacceptable to me. But even more importantly, my health and peace of mind wouldn't be nearly as good as they are today if I had settled for passive reliance on a pill to solve my problem.

Testing for Testosterone

When I read or hear about something I think can help me be more vigorous or virile or healthy, I always make a practice of asking my doctor what he knows about it. Sometimes, he knows a little. Sometimes he knows a lot. And sometimes what he knows has a profound effect on my well being and my whole approach to life.

I can't think of a better example of this than the day I asked my doctor about testosterone injections after reading about them in a magazine.

Have you ever heard of testosterone? Do you know what it is and what it does? If not, it's high time you found out – especially if you're one of those people who attributes his (or her) loss of interest in sex to advancing age. I guarantee your doctor knows about testosterone and what it may be able to do for you. But the chances are, he'll never say a word about it – unless you ask.

Testosterone is a male hormone released by the testes and adrenal glands and circulated in the bloodstream. In a manner of speaking, it is to men what the female hormone estrogen is to women. It could be called the essence of maleness and of the male sex drive. A high testosterone level is what gives many young "studs" in their teens and early 20s an almost limitless appetite for sexual adventure. And, conversely, declining testosterone in older men is what makes them lose interest in sex.

Your testosterone level can easily be determined by a simple blood test (but the odds are 99 out of 100 that you'll have to request the test on your own; it isn't part of any standard physical exam, as far as I know). When the test scores are in, the problem usually becomes obvious immediately. Those randy young "studs" will show an average serum testosterone level of about 800, while the typical guy of 55 or 60 will "flunk out" with a level below 200 – often way below.

More Than a Sex Stimulant

The thing is, your doctor can go beyond merely testing your testosterone; he can also increase your level with periodic injections. I've monitored my own testosterone level for years, and I've gotten to the point where I can tell if it's low even before the test is run. When it is, an injection quickly counteracts the problem. The beneficial effects of one shot will often last for up to two or three months.

Because of my personal experience with testosterone, I've become convinced that it's much more than a mere stimulant for your sex life. In addition, I believe the lack of it in older males may be a primary key to the overall aging process. Besides boosting libido and sexual performance, this "youth hormone" also promotes muscle growth, bone strength and a healthy arterial system.

Recently, when I went too long between injections, my testosterone level fell to about 150, and I experienced some very disturbing symptoms. My body fat, which usually runs around 8 percent, suddenly went up, and my lean muscle mass went down. I felt temporarily as if I had aged several years overnight. I don't intend to let it fall that low again.

Anyone can have his testosterone checked regularly and keep its level regulated. There's nothing illegal or even immoral about testosterone shots. Even women can sometimes benefit from testosterone, but since it's a male hormone, extra care should be exercised in giving it to females. It can stimulate hair growth and other male characteristics.

If in doubt – do I have to say it again? – ask your doctor!

Why Women Need Estrogen

Diminishing interest in sex and a loss of libido aren't exclusively a male problem by any means. In many respects, the hormone estrogen, produced by the ovaries, is to femininity what testosterone is to masculinity. It is a necessary component of proper sexual function. It is also much, much more.

Typically, a woman's estrogen level remains constant, except for normal fluctuations during the mentrual cycle, from the time she's about 13 until she's in her late 30s. But beginning around age 40, most women's bodies no longer produce enough estrogen. The resulting shortage of estrogen can trigger a host of physical disorders and sudden aging. It can also set the stage for severe health complications in years to come.

Here's the problem – one that affects many women in their 40s and early 50s: It's generally recognized by the medical profession that women who have passed through menopause or had hysterectomies that resulted in "surgical menopause" need estrogen replacement therapy (ERT) to protect them against cardiovascular disease. But few doctors routinely prescribe estrogen for pre-menopausal women who still have their ovaries.

Since the average age for menopause is about 51, this means there's often a gap of up to a dozen years during which a woman's natural estrogen production falls sharply but nothing is usually done to replace it. This can lead to major problems, including premature aging, a loss of sexuality, increased risk of developing such diseases as osteoporosis, colon cancer and Alzheimer's Disease, not to mention a heightening of the "hot flashes" and volatile mood swings associated with approaching menopause. And without enough estrogen, one thing is certain – a woman's sex life will wither and die.

If you're a woman in her 40s and 50s and you aren't taking estrogen, it's high time you asked your doctor about it. While some studies show a link between estrogen replacement therapy and an increased risk of breast cancer, many doctors are outspokenly skeptical of these reports. As one Dallas gynecologist told me bluntly: "I see no evidence in my patients of any increased incidence or increased risk of cancer."

Something else you may want to ask your doctor about is the possibility of receiving a different kind of estrogen instead of the once-a-day Premarin tablets that most physicians routinely prescribe. Premarin is manufactured from the urine of pregnant mares (that's where the name comes from) and a growing number of gynecologists feel that substituting human estrogen for Premarin will not only do the same job better but also reduce any attendant health risks.

Unfortunately, there is currently no mass-produced estrogen tablet containing the human hormone. Apparently, the FDA doesn't think such a pill is necessary. But some gynecologists have teamed up with pharmacists to prescribe and produce human-estrogen gels and implantable pellets. The pellets, which last for three months, appear to be especially effective.

I'll have more to say about the sexual implications of estrogen replacement therapy in a later chapter. But for now the important thing to understand is that if you're a woman of 40 or over, you'll be doing yourself a tremendous favor by asking your doctor about its potential benefits for you. If you start on estrogen now, you may be able to avoid all or most of the tormenting symptoms so often associated with menopause.

In fact, some doctors go so far as to say you may be able to avoid menopause itself. Dr. Robert A. Wilson, a prominent New York gynecologist, was quoted in a recent *Time* article as saying that "menopause is unnecessary. It can be prevented entirely."

Whether you believe it or not, it's certainly something to think about.

Don't Be Afraid to Ask

The Bible says, "Ask and ye shall receive." I believe it. I've never been reticent about asking for information. That's how I've learned a large percentage of what I know. And there's no more important area in which to put this approach to work than in matters pertaining to your own health and longevity.

I've asked doctors questions on every conceivable subject related to medicine – everything from human growth hormone to chelation therapy to penile implants. They haven't always provided clearcut answers, but they've certainly broadened my understanding and helped me make more informed decisions about matters that affect me.

Doctors, of course, are only human. As such, they are fallible like the rest of us. They do make mistakes sometimes, and they don't always have all the answers. But if you're a patient – and all of us are at one time or another – you can only gain by plugging into their superior knowledge.

If your physician isn't open and candid with you – if he doesn't answer your legitimate questions forthrightly and to the best of his ability, then you probably need to look for another doctor.

The Heart of the Matter

New drugs, new procedures and new forms of therapy come into the "medical marketplace" with dizzying speed these days. Probably not any one doctor is familiar with all of them. But any specialist who stays current in his specialty should have a good grasp of what's happening in his own field.

In cardiology, for example, many exciting, life-extending developments are taking place. Researchers have learned that something as simple as taking a single aspirin tablet a day can greatly reduce the risk of heart attacks. And a Scandinavian study of the cholesterol-lowering drug simvastatin showed that it reduced the risk of coronary death among patients with previous histories of severe heart and artery disease by 42 percent.

To leaders in heart disease research, the success of simvastatin and similar drugs has virtually ended once and for all the debate over whether controlling cholesterol can effectively prevent heart attacks. Clearly, it can – and does.

Yet as of now, the vast majority of patients who have already had heart attacks or bypass surgery or angioplasty still aren't receiving any of these cholesterol-lowering agents. And in all probability it will take several years for most patients to start benefitting from these drugs. In the meantime, millions of people will die unnecessarily.

Cardiovascular disease is the world's number-one killer. Cancers of all types run a distant second. An estimated 12 million people will die of coronary disease this year. A fourth of all the people now living on earth are projected to become victims of heart and artery disease. But many of these grim statistics could be changed, if more people asked their doctors more questions – and then actively used the answers for their own benefit.

If you have high cholesterol that hasn't responded to diet, weight loss, exercise or other lifestyle changes, asking your doctor about one of the "statin" drugs could be the most important question of your life.

In fact, your life could well depend on it.

Surgery Offers Options

Many people have a consuming, deep-seated fear of surgery – "going under the knife," as it's still sometimes called. For some, it represents the ultimate medical nightmare. But I'm very fortunate in this regard. I've been able to look at surgery as just one more option, one more weapon in my personal arsenal against aging.

One advantage I have is that I've never been afraid of a surgical procedure (which is a good thing, since I've undergone over a dozen of them). Another is that I heal with such remarkable speed that the surgeon himself often has a hard time believing it. There have been times when I underwent surgery in the morning and was actually in the gym working out that same evening.

Admittedly, I've never experienced anything as serious as open-heart surgery or surgery to remove a tumor, and I fervently hope I never do. But for me, surgeries that many other people would do almost anything to avoid have become a standard means to an end for me.

In almost two decades of professional wrestling, I suffered a wide range of injuries that can only be corrected by surgery. Just recently, I finished up a round of operations designed to correct nerve damage in my shoulders, wrists and elbows. Now that it's out of the way, I'll be able to work out more vigorously – as well as more comfortably – and get myself in the best shape I've ever been in. For me, these surgeries were a vehicle to better health and a more active life, a minor inconvenience that I gladly accepted in order to achieve a greater goal.

But I wonder how many other guys in their 60s would seriously consider four different "non-essential" operations in a single four-month period just to get rid of some nagging discomforts they'd been living with for years. Not too many, I'd guess. And I probably wouldn't have, either, except for one thing:

I asked my doctor (in this case, my surgeon) about it!

As a result, I learned about surgical procedures that could correct my problems, most of them procedures that were developed and perfected long after I incurred those problems in the first place.

Surgery is yet another medical discipline where tremendous innovations have taken place in recent years. Modern surgery is actually many specialties lumped together under one broad heading – neurosurgery, orthopedic surgery, cardiovascular surgery, reconstructive surgery, cosmetic surgery and so forth.

Nothing can make you feel older than hobbling around on a bum knee that you hurt playing high school football 30 or 40 years ago. At the time of your injury, maybe you were told there was nothing to be done, that you'd simply have to put up with periodic pain and discomfort the rest of your life. But with the great recent advances in sports medicine and orthoscopic surgery, this may no longer be true.

    The point is, you'll never know if you don't ask.

"If I had another face to wear, do you think I would wear this one?"
—ABRAHAM LINCOLN

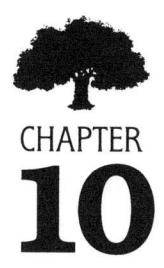

CHAPTER 10

Plastic and Cosmetic Surgery – What to Expect

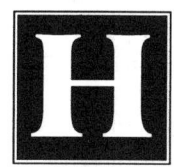

How many of your personal friends and acquaintances have had a facelift? A "nose job"? A "tummy tuck"? Breast augmentation (or reduction)?

For most Americans, the answer to these questions ranges from "Very few" to "None at all." And even if you know a few people whom you suspect of having had one of these procedures done, chances are they don't make a habit of discussing it, and, of course, you don't want to be nosy.

Now let me ask you another question: Have you ever thought – even for just a brief moment or two – about hiring a plastic surgeon to correct certain flaws in your own face or body?

Hey, quit blushing! Your secret's safe with me. I won't tell a soul.

As enlightened as we've become in many areas, it's hard for me to understand why so many people – especially men – continue to attach such a taboo to cosmetic surgery. To a majority of the general public, it's still a practice reserved for a few over-the-hill actresses and eccentric socialites. It's still the subject of a lot of snickering and speculation at cocktail parties.

You know the kind of thing I mean. A busty young lady in a low-cut dress walks past a group of guys, and one of them winks and whispers: "I wonder how much of that's silicone and how much of it's real."

Or some saggy dowager eyes an attractive middle-aged lady whose youthful face belies her years and mutters enviously: "If she has one more facelift, her cheeks are going to end up above her eyebrows!"

The Joke May Be on You

Despite our acceptance of many modern social and scientific innovations, surgery performed strictly to enhance one's physical appearance remains something of a national joke.

Well, if you're 50 or over, I suggest you quit laughing. In all probability, the joke may be on you.

As Dr. George A. Toledo, an exceptionally skilled plastic surgeon in Dallas, Texas, who has performed several cosmetic procedures on me, puts it: "There are basically very few people who couldn't benefit from plastic surgery. For people 50 or older, in particular, age has usually taken its toll on their appearance. Many of them could take 20 or more years off their looks by having these conditions corrected surgically."

Many of the flaws that plastic surgery can remove, of course, have nothing to do with age. It's not unusual for younger people also to be unhappy with some aspect of their appearance. Some recent surveys show that 60 million Americans don't like their chins, that 6 million don't like their eyes, and that up to 40 percent would give their bodies a grade of no better than a "C." For all these reasons, plastic surgery is winning greater and greater acceptance. Despite the fact that the average person is still resistant to the idea, hundreds of thousands of men and women will undergo cosmetic surgery this year. And when they see the results, most of them will be very glad they did.

How to Lose 20 Years

By the time I was approaching 60, my body was as fit as ever and my skeletal muscles as firm and well-toned as they had been when I was 30. But I had to admit that a few other areas could stand some improvement.

I talked to Dr. Toledo about what could be done to correct these problems, and he made several recommendations. One of my most obvious trouble spots was my nose, which had been repeatedly battered and broken by thousands of pro wrestling bouts. Fixing my nose was more than a matter of cosmetics, he explained. It was also a matter of getting enough air through my nostrils. During surgery, Dr. Toledo had to break my nose four times to straighten it. But when he was done, I not only looked a lot better, but I could also breathe through my nose for the first time in 40 years.

On average, it takes two weeks for a person's appearance to return to normal after plastic surgery. But because I heal so quickly, I was back in circulation within about a week, and nobody knew what had happened. My friends and associates immediately noticed a difference in the way I looked, but they really couldn't tell what caused it. "Wow, Ray, you really look great," they'd say. "What did you do to yourself?"

I grinned and said, "Oh, I just lost a few pounds, that's all."

Plastic surgery has come a tremendously long way since it was first used to repair the disfiguring injuries of World War II veterans. Nowadays, for instance, the scar tissue from a facelift – what little there is of it – can usually be confined to the inside of the ear or hidden under the hairline, where it's virtually invisible. And liposuction causes only temporary bruising and leaves no lasting marks. Unless you want to tell people you've had plastic surgery, there's really no need for them to know.

A properly performed facelift could take at least 20 years off your appearance. This means if you're 60, you'll look about 40 after the surgery. For the average person, the beneficial effects should last up to 20 years, maybe more. But if you want to continue to look "forty-something," a facelift may be required every 7 to 10 years.

Men Get Into the Act

Most cosmetic surgeries are still performed on women. At last count, female patients outnumbered males by more than five to one. But the number of male patients is growing. In 1990, about 16 percent of all facial cosmetic surgery patients were men. The procedure they requested most was nose contouring, followed by eyelid surgery, fat suction and facelifts.

One reason that men from every walk of life are choosing cosmetic surgery is today's youth-oriented society. But an even more practical reason is the competitiveness of today's job market. When a man has bags under his eyes or a double chin or a pot belly, it can affect his business dealings and his ability to get a better job. Studies have repeatedly shown that better looking candidates get better jobs, all other things being equal.

Men whose advancement and earning capabilities depend heavily on first impressions are among the likeliest candidates for cosmetic surgery.

Traditionally, many men don't care that much about how they look, but those who have a definite goal in mind often do. When you have 20 guys competing for the same vice-president's position, for example, it shouldn't come as any surprise that the one who looks the best usually gets the job. A man's profession or vocation also plays a part. A salesman is much more likely than a mechanic to get a facelift.

Other men decide to have plastic surgery after observing the good results it produced in their wives or girlfriends.

Goodbye Flab, Hello Muscles

Liposuction has become a major weapon in the female gender's ongoing war against flab. Not surprisingly, this technique of sucking fat cells out of thighs, bottoms, waistlines and other portions of the body tops the list of the most popular procedures performed by modern plastic surgeons. And it's a prime example of the technological advancements that have been achieved in cosmetic surgery over the past 15 years or so.

While it's not really recommended as a weight-reduction measure, liposuction can remove up to 10 quarts of fat cells in one operation, which can result in a significant loss of weight. The procedure used to be stopped after removing about two quarts because of attendant blood loss, but new techniques allow much more fat to be removed in a single procedure.

The greatest benefits of liposuction are the improvements it can make in body contour. The ideal candidate for liposuction isn't the 300-pounder who wants to get down to 275 without having to diet or exercise, but the person who is 5 or 10 or 20 pounds overweight with stubborn bulges of fatty tissue in certain areas of the body. It can "sculpt" the body and emphasize muscle structures that have been obscured by fat.

Even many fit individuals still have double chins, "love handles" at their waists or little pooches of fat somewhere else that mar their otherwise trim appearance. As I've often remarked to people I was training: "There's no such thing as spot reducing through exercise. You can firm and tone the muscles in any part of the body, and you can lower your total body fat through a combination of exercise and proper nutrition. But regardless of what you've read or heard, exercise alone can't 'burn off' fat in a given area."

Some localized fat deposits are the results of genetics or aging, and once they're there, no amount of aerobics or fasting will get rid of them completely.

Liposuction is a viable answer to that problem, however, and one that more and more people are taking advantage of.

Perfecting the Female Breast

No object in human culture draws more attention than the female breast. From a male viewpoint, breast size and shape are key measurements of feminine glamor and sex appeal. To women, breasts often have an even deeper psychological significance relating to self-concept and self-esteem.

Unfortunately, few women are endowed with perfect breasts, and even for the few that are, the impact of pregnancy and childbirth, losing or gaining weight and simple aging can cause many problems as the years go by.

Fortunately, however, plastic surgery now offers more options than ever before for women who are unhappy with their breasts. Nowhere does modern medical science work greater marvels than in correcting the various imperfections of nature that affect the female breast.

There are many procedures that can be done on breasts. Most women want larger ones, but breast reduction is also common. So are procedures to lift, shape and reduce nipple size.

The most common and simplest procedure is enlargement or enhancement. In medical terms, the procedure is called augmentation mammaplasty. It involves inserting an implant made of silicone rubber and filled with silicone gel, a saline solution or a combination of the two. Other new types of filler material are also being developed. Currently, however, the FDA allows only saline-filled implants to be used in this country for cosmetic breast augmentation.

The implant is positioned directly beneath the nipple, and may be placed either directly behind the breast tissue or underneath the chest muscle. Many plastic surgeons favor the under-the-muscle placement for two main reasons: One, it may reduce the chances of the most common problem associated with implants – a condition called capsular contracture, in which a capsule of scar tissue forms around the implant, squeezing it and causing it to contract until the breast feels unnaturally firm. Two, it may also make it easier to examine the breasts for cancer using mammography. Other surgeons endorse the over-the-muscle position because it causes less post-operative discomfort and may produce a better cosmetic result. Any woman considering breast enhancement surgery should receive a detailed explanation of these options from her surgeon.

Recent studies show, by the way, that silicone breast implants have no harmful effects on the immune system and are not responsible for causing any diseases in humans. No relationship has been found between silicone implants and breast cancer. Women who have implants are no more likely to contract breast cancer than those who don't.

Other plastic surgical procedures for the breasts, such as a breast lift or breast reduction, are much more complex than breast enlargement. Breast reduction, in particular, is classified as major reconstructive surgery. Most women who undergo it do so more for physical relief from the discomforts associated with oversize breasts than for cosmetic improvement.

Because so many psychological and symbolic factors are involved in altering the physical appearance of the breasts, a bond of trust and understanding between patient and surgeon is especially essential when plastic surgery on the breasts is being considered. Most plastic surgeons prefer that husbands or life partners of prospective patients be included in pre-surgery consultations.

"Make sure you understand the procedure and what to expect from it," Dr. Toledo says. "And no woman should let herself be pushed into having any breast procedure if she has misgivings. She needs to be certain that she personally wants it and isn't doing it just to please someone else."

Hair-Raising Experiences

The steady improvements in surgical hair-replacement techniques should be of special interest to men. Most of the more than 40 million American males who are affected by male-pattern baldness can be helped significantly by one or more of the following procedures:

– Punch grafts are the most commonly used technique. Round plugs, each measuring about one-eighth of an inch in diameter and containing about 15 hairs, are taken from a donor site at the back of the scalp and fitted into holes punched in a bald area. About 50 grafts can be made in one session, and it usually takes several sessions spaced several months apart to fill in the targeted area.

– These larger plugs can now be augmented by "miniplugs" about half their size or even smaller "microplugs," which are used to fill in spaces between the larger plugs and add some natural-looking irregularity to the hairline. This technique prevents the appearance of orderly "corn rows" frequently associated with a bad hair transplant.

– Strip grafts are like punch grafts, but are long and thin rather than round. They measure up to a quarter-inch wide and two inches long and are frequently used to finish the hairline after a bald spot is filled in with plugs.

– Flaps are used to eliminate large bald areas at the front of the head. Sections of hair-bearing scalp are removed from a donor site, but left connected to the original site at one end, then swiveled to cover the bald spot. The improvement is immediate and dramatic.

– The quickest way to reduce large areas of baldness on the crown of the head is called "scalp reduction." A section of bald skin measuring one to two inches wide by as much as six or seven inches long is cut out of the scalp, and the two sides of the opening are then pulled together and sutured closed.

The results of hair-replacement surgery are permanent and can be remarkable. The biggest drawback is the time required – typically 18 months or longer. But with patience, the rewards can be great.

Looking at Other Options

There are many other cosmetic surgery procedures that can improve appearance and combat the effects of aging. Our purpose here isn't to discuss all of them in detail, but merely to provide an overview of the possibilities and some general information about a few of the most effective and popular.

A total rejuvenation of an aging face, for instance, may include not only a facelift, but a browlift, eyelid surgery, nose reshaping, a chin implant and a chemical skin peel or dermabrasion. Which procedures and how many of them you elect to have done will depend on the signs of aging you see in your own face and how much they bother you.

People in their 50s and 60s may require lift surgery to get rid of sagging excess skin on the abdomen, thighs, buttocks or arms after an extreme weight loss or following liposuction. Such lift procedures as tummy tucks are widely used because the results are dramatic and the scars can be covered by a bikini. Arm or thigh tucks can leave visible scars, but sometimes there's no other way to fix the problem.

Many women in their 40s, 50s and 60s have periodic injections of fat cells and collagen to tighten and "freshen" their skin or plump their lips. Often, they'll come in for an injection just before a big social event. The effects of collagen are only temporary, usually lasting from a few days to a few weeks at most, and surgeons caution that no one should expect permanent or long-term improvement from these injections. Fat transfer, on the other hand, has been shown to be longlasting.

Cigarette smokers face special difficulties during and after plastic surgery, because nicotine causes shrinkage in the small blood vessels all over their bodies. Particularly in procedures involving elevating skin flaps, in which the blood supply to an area is interrupted, smokers can experience skin loss, slow healing and poor scarring.

Most plastic surgeons recommend that if a patient can't quit smoking completely, he or she should at least stop temporarily for several weeks, and some surgeons refuse to do surgery on smokers at all, especially facelifts, tummy tucks and breast reductions.

How Much Does it Cost?

Even for people who seriously consider cosmetic surgery, there are often two primary obstacles that keep them from actually going ahead with it. The first of these is financial. If you've never had any experience with cosmetic surgery, you probably think of it as being very expensive. It isn't cheap, but you may be pleasantly surprised at how affordable it can be.

Take a facelift, for example. The surgeon's fee generally ranges from $4,000 to $7,000, not including anesthesia or a stay in the hospital. While this is a considerable amount, it's less than half what most people spend for a new automobile – and the "new face" that results from this surgery will still be looking good long after that car's worn out.

The following are some other ballpark figures for various types of plastic surgery. (Again, the cost for anesthesia, operating room or hospital stay, if needed, aren't included.)

Surgical fees for breast enlargement range from $1,000 to $5,500. Breast lift surgery runs from $1,000 to $6,000, and breast reduction surgery runs from $1,500 to $8,000. Surgical fees for liposuction range from $500 to $5,000, depending on how much fat is removed and how many areas of the body are treated. Sometimes, secondary touchups, if needed, are included in the overall fee.

Surgeons charge from $2,500 to $8,500 for an abdominoplasty or tummy tuck. The fee for a chemical peel and dermabrasion ranges from $100 to $3,000, depending on whether the procedure involves one small area or the whole face. And hair replacement grafts cost $15 to $60 per plug, meaning that an average transplant of 50 plugs will cost $750 to $3,000. A strip graft costs an average of $400, and scalp reduction and flap procedures run from $1,000 to $3,000. Blepharoplasty or eyelid surgery costs from $1,000 to $3,500 for two lids or from $1,500 to $5,000 for all four. The fee for rhinoplasty or a nose job varies widely -- from $1,500 to $6,000, depending on the length and complexity of the surgery.

People usually have the idea that plastic surgery is more expensive than it really is. Although most procedures aren't covered by insurance, financing is usually available, and many surgeons also accept credit cards.

The point is, plastic surgery is no longer a luxury reserved for the very rich. In fact, more than six out of every 10 people who have cosmetic surgery have family incomes of $50,000 a year or less.

Overcoming Your Fears

The other major obstacle that causes many people to shy away from cosmetic surgery is fear of the unknown.

Many people are afraid of doctors in general. Others are terrified of the idea of being cut. Put these together and you have a truly formidable deterrent to seeking the kind of help that plastic surgery offers.

The best way to overcome this fear is to talk to a plastic surgeon and get a complete explanation of what's involved in the surgery you're contemplating – costs, recovery time, the amount of discomfort and scarring to expect, and the realistic limitations on what can be accomplished surgically. It may be wise to consult more than one surgeon to make sure you find the right one for you.

It's only natural for the patient to wonder if the surgeon's going to do a good job, and it's up to the surgeon to win the patient's trust. Sometimes, surgeons point out, people are more nervous when the surgery is elective than they would be if it were dictated by some medical condition. If someone's having a tumor removed, the patient figures he or she has no choice in the matter. But when the surgery is cosmetic in nature, the same patient may think, "I don't have to have this done. Maybe I shouldn't."

It Can Be Habit-Forming

Based on my own experience, as well as my observations of other people, it can be hard to talk yourself into having your first cosmetic procedure done. After you see the results, though, it gets much easier.

Sometimes, in fact, it gets too easy. Some people who can afford it get to the point of wanting every single one of their physical flaws corrected by surgery. They get the idea that more is better, and it becomes an obsession. They start badgering their surgeons to suction this and lift that and restructure something else. I've known individuals who'd have a facelift every three or four years if they could find a surgeon to do it.

Getting too many facelifts can cause serious scarring and damage your looks, rather than enhance them. But when you start expecting a facelift to work miracles in your life, the biggest danger can be psychological. No kind of cosmetic surgery will keep your husband from playing around with his secretary or your wife from having an affair. People who think it will may need counselling more than they need another facelift.

Plastic surgery can, however, increase your self-esteem, make you more outgoing and assertive, and even change your personality for the better.

There's No Reason to Wait

It would be awfully nice if a person of 50 or 60 could walk into a plastic surgeon's office, lay a photograph of himself at age 35 on the doctor's desk, and say "Make me look just like this again" with every confidence that the surgeon could do exactly that.

Someday in the future, this may fall into the realm of possibility, but it won't happen anytime soon. The advancements in plastic surgery over the past decade or two have made amazing transformations possible, but there are limits and there probably always will be.

"There's no doubt we'll continue to see innovations in the future," says Dr. Toledo, "but it will be hard to match the progress of the past 10 to 15 years. Right now, we're closing in on perfection where our surgical results are concerned, and it's very difficult to get from 90 percent of perfection to 100 percent."

In other words, there's no reason to wait for something better to come along. The plastic surgeon's skills are at an all-time peak right now. There isn't likely to be a better time in the foreseeable future to make maximum use of those skills.

Every bit as important as the new look produced by the surgery itself are the direct and indirect spinoff benefits that it can set in motion.

It's not unusual for a facelift or some other anti-aging procedure to give a person a whole new lease on life. When you look in the mirror each day and see a sagging, wrinkled face looking back at you, it can't help but give you a tired, dispirited, negative feeling about yourself. But when you see that face change to resemble the mental image you still have of yourself as a young, newly mature person, it can make a profound difference in how you think of yourself.

One Man's Transformation

In addition to the visible signs of aging, our 50s and 60s are also often a time of mental, emotional and psychological stress. A friend of mine – I'll call him Dave – was beset by a grinding series of setbacks, misfortunes and unwelcome changes within one five-year period beginning when he was 54. His parents died within two years of each other; his son became a drug abuser and dropped out of college; he lost his $60,000-a-year job and the only new one he could find paid a much lower salary; and he and his wife began to have problems.

Dave looked terrible and seemed to feel even worse. He was still in his 50s, but he looked like a man of 70 or more. There were big bags under his eyes and folds of loose skin around his neck. His eyelids drooped to the point that he looked as if he was half-asleep all the time. He was severely depressed and withdrawn. He broke off contact with most of his friends.

But for his 60th birthday, Dave gave himself a special birthday present – a facelift and eyelid surgery, which turned back the clock for him. Suddenly, he saw a different guy looking back at him from the mirror, a guy who looked more like 40 than 60 and one Dave had almost forgotten existed.

Dave's state of mind improved overnight. He started an exercise program, began to take an interest in nutrition, even went out and bought some sporty new clothes to replace the drab suits he had worn for so long. As he regained his stamina and his interest in life, he started taking his wife out to dinner and the theatre two or three times a week. Pretty soon, they were having so much fun together that their marital problems were all forgotten.

The last time I saw Dave, he looked, literally, like a new man. He sounded like one, too. "I feel great," he said. "For a long time I felt like I was walking around with one foot in the grave, but now I'm back in the world again."

Plastic surgery alone didn't accomplish this incredible change in Dave. But it was the catalyst. It provided the psychological boost he needed to get him started in the right direction.

I believe it can serve the same purpose for many people.

A Few Words of Caution

As I'm sure you can tell by now, I'm sold on cosmetic surgery as another invaluable tool to fight aging. In the future, I won't hesitate to take advantage of other procedures that can help my appearance and the way I feel about myself.

But it's definitely not a decision to be made lightly, and I do want to offer a few words of caution.

If you're contemplating a cosmetic procedure, I strongly recommend that you rely on the training and skill of one of the 4,000-plus board-certified plastic surgeons practicing in this country. Other types of physicians and surgeons also perform cosmetic surgery, but many of them are dermatologists or even ear, nose and throat doctors, and they lack the background and expertise of true plastic surgeons.

(Plastic surgery, incidentally, has nothing to do with plastic – that tough, stretchy material we encounter in a hundred different forms each day. The surgical term comes from the Greek word "plastikos," which refers to "molding" or "shaping," which is, of course, what a plastic surgeon does.)

Some of these other cosmetic surgeons may offer much lower prices than those charged by real plastic surgeons, but the savings could turn out to be a very costly form of false economy.

In one respect, cosmetic surgery is very much like other products and services. Generally, you get what you pay for. If a doctor has to discount his rates, there's always a reason, so when fees seem extremely low, my advice is "Beware."

Much has been made of laser surgery in the past few years, and some cosmetic surgeons promote this technique as being faster, easier and causing less post-operative swelling and discomfort. But the truth is, a laser is simply another cutting tool, and offers no appreciable advantage over a scalpel in most cosmetic procedures.

"A laser is somewhat better for removing birthmarks, tattoos and other surface skin blemishes," says Dr. Toledo. "Otherwise, the idea that it produces superior results is mostly a gimmick."

If you want to find out more about specific surgical procedures, costs, recovery times, potential problems and what results to expect, I urge you to read a book entitled *Guide to Cosmetic Surgery*, written by Josleen Wilson. It's endorsed by the American Society of Plastic and Reconstructive Surgeons and it can tell you most of what you need to know.

And if you decide to go ahead with it, what will friends and acquaintances in your age group say? In most cases, not a word.

They may be green with envy and consumed by curiosity, but they'll probably be too self-conscious to come right out and ask: "Hey, why do you look so much younger than I do?"

*"We drink to on another's health
and spoil our own."*
–JEROME K. JEROME

CHAPTER 11

Booze and Recreational Drugs– Are They Worth It?

As far as I know, no one's ever called me a prude or accused me of being a "killjoy" or a "wet blanket." I've always subscribed to the belief that life was meant to be full and enjoyable, and I haven't regretted partaking of many of the worldly pleasures this existence has to offer.

I've also never believed in preaching to people or making lofty moral judgments concerning their habits and lifestyles. My motto is "Live and let live." For that reason, what I'm about to say in this chapter may come as a surprise to some of my long-time friends and acquaintances.

But the inescapable fact is, heavy alcohol consumption and/or the habitual use of so-called "recreational drugs" such as cocaine, marijuana, amphetamines and other illegal substances is simply incompatible with a long, healthy, satisfying life. If you want to make a steady practice of getting sloshed or stoned, that's your business. When you do, though, you should be aware that you're making a major tradeoff. It comes down to swapping vigorous, productive years of life for a fleeting "high," a fuzzy head and the potential for truly serious health problems.

Please understand, I'm not saying that anybody who drinks or does drugs automatically forfeits the chance to live to a ripe old age. We've all heard stories about some legendary character who drank a quart of whiskey every day and still made it into his 90s. Somewhere, there may be a hardy centenarian who fires up a joint every hour on the hour and snorts a few lines of coke each morning before breakfast. There are exceptions to every rule, but they are exceptions.

What I'm saying is that the odds of enjoying a second healthy 50 years are overwhelmingly in favor of people who (a) scrupulously avoid illicit drugs, and (b) either abstain totally from alcohol or limit themselves to no more than a couple of drinks a day.

If you've reached your 50th birthday, or if you soon will, it's time to weigh your own odds.

A Spreading Epidemic

Never having used recreational drugs myself, I find it impossible to understand the aura that makes these addictive, outlawed, dangerous substances so popular among well-educated, financially favored and seemingly successful people.

When I was a teenager in the 1940s and '50s, the sidewalks of New York were already littered with pushers and junkies. Although at that time the "drug culture" had yet to invade mid-America, heroin, marijuana and other drugs could be bought on every other street corner in my native Brooklyn. But the people who sought and used these drugs were universally regarded as misfits, losers and criminal scum. Decent people never dreamed of smoking a reefer or injecting "horse" into their veins. Those who did were objects of derision and disgust. We called them "dope fiends."

Because of this, I grew up with the firm conviction that only the most ignorant, poverty-ridden, hopeless, twisted people used dope. This class of people still does constitute the biggest market for illicit drugs, but over the past 20 years or so, an insidious epidemic of habitual drug abuse has spread through all layers of our society.

In the process, a deeply disturbing – and to me unexplainable – trend has become apparent across this country. Many of the most flagrant abusers of controlled substances are now the very people who would seem to have the least possible reason to use them – acclaimed actors and actresses, noted artists, powerful political leaders, young athletes at the peak of their careers, ultra-wealthy business tycoons, highly respected doctors and lawyers, even ministers and educators.

The more I think about this, the less sense it makes. How otherwise intelligent, knowledgeable, worldly, successful, admired people can let themselves be caught in this trap is beyond my comprehension.

The one thing I do know, however, is why I never tried cocaine or other recreational drugs. If the stuff makes normally sane people feel so euphoric that they're willing to throw away everything for it – including their own lives – then I'm sure I'd love it so much I'd be hooked immediately. I think of myself as being a pretty strong person, but I have enough sense to know I can't fight something like that and win. The only safe route is strict avoidance. So my choice has been to forego the pleasure entirely and never to take that first step. I've never regretted for a moment making that choice and sticking with it.

Killer With a Capital "C"

Obviously, though, if you have experimented with drugs at some point in your life – or if you still do – you can't help but approach the problem from a different perspective than mine. I've heard drug users say, "Oh, it's no worse than a lot of other habits; it's just that it's against the law."

This may be true. Cigarette smoking, for example, is perfectly legal, yet every sane adult knows it kills people. So does alcohol abuse and overeating. Any destructive habit does damage that, over time, may be impossible to repair, and in that sense, drug abuse should be viewed in the same way as other destructive habits.

There are people who smoke only two or three cigarettes a day, but there are far more who smoke two or three packs a day. When does a bad habit become a dependency? An addiction?

If you have an actual drug dependency, I'd recommend getting professional help at the earliest possible moment. You can begin by making an appointment with your doctor and laying your cards on the table. Whatever steps may be necessary beyond that, I'd urge you to take them with the goal of getting drug-free and staying that way.

Even long-term addictions can be broken. It happens every day. It's never too late, but the older you get, the higher the stakes become. This isn't morality or legality talking. It's common sense.

Don't con yourself into thinking what you're doing won't hurt you. Some drugs, like cocaine, are killers. Extensive research into the effects of "nose candy" show you don't have to take an overdose for the stuff to have lethal consequences. While you're feeling the rush of euphoria that comes with the first snort or two, your blood pressure and heart rate are soaring, and the risk of blowing out an artery in your brain and suffering a fatal or crippling stroke is magnified many times over. So is your risk of heart attack.

This happens every time you take a sniff of coke. These very same effects have struck down young, superbly conditioned athletes in their 20s. One moment, they were full of life and excitement, on the brink of vast wealth, glory and public adulation. The next moment, they were dead forever.

Presumably, you're not nearly as young as they were. Probably, you're not as physically fit, either. Think about it.

A Master of Deception

Cocaine is also a master of deceit and deception. I've had users tell me how much it heightened their sexual arousal and lowered the inhibitions of their partners, but based on every authoritative piece of information I can find, this is nothing more than a dope dream.

In reality, cocaine more often renders men incapable of performing sexually. It turns sex into a spectator sport, rather than a participation sport. But it may fuzz a person's perception sufficiently to make him think he's taking part in some sort of wild orgy, when, in fact, he's merely watching from the sidelines. Most of the time, the only sexual activity any man's likely to engage in while under the influence of cocaine is what I jokingly refer to as "oral sex" – the kind you talk about later without actually remembering.

While many users also claim that marijuana adds to their enjoyment of sex, the lethargy-producing, mildly hallucinogenic qualities of the drug leave this very much open for debate. In actuality, I suspect many people who try to make love after smoking a few joints have a strong tendency to fall asleep during the sex act.

These days, marijuana is considered so mild and relatively innocuous in comparison with "hard drugs" that its chances for eventual legalization appear to be improving every year. But is marijuana harmless from a health standpoint? Don't you believe it!

Much research still needs to be carried out on the subject, but virtually all the studies done to date into the effects of "loco weed" on human health show marijuana smoke to be many times more damaging to the lungs and cardiovascular system than ordinary tobacco smoke. In addition to the medical problems it can cause, marijuana is every bit as dangerous as alcohol when someone under its influence gets behind the wheel of a car.

The point is, what's the point? If you've reached the age of 50 or so without ever trying recreational drugs, there's absolutely no valid reason to start now. If you've had occasional past encounters with illegal substances, it's time to charge off these experiences to the impetuous foolishness of youth and forget about them.

And if you have an actual dependency problem, it's time to admit it and get the help you need.

Recreational drugs and good health after 50 are simply incompatible. They don't go together and they never will. If you choose the short-lived highs you get from drugs over the long-term natural high you get from being physically fit, mentally alert and in charge of your life, so be it.

But if you get shortchanged in the tradeoff, you've got no complaints coming later.

Saying Goodbye to Booze

On the subject of drugs, I'm forced to rely on what I've read, heard and observed as a non-participant. But when it comes to booze, I can speak from extensive personal experience.

In other words, I'm not writing this from the perspective of a lifelong teetotaller. On the contrary, for most of my adult life, I was an almost-daily drinker. Being able to buy, serve and consume alcoholic beverages was one of the symbols of the "good life" to which I had aspired as a youngster. But I also liked the taste of the stuff – especially scotch. I never thought of myself as having a "drinking problem," yet like most people who imbibe regularly, I occasionally overdid it and ended up with a hangover or some other unpleasant after-effect.

I can remember looking at myself in the mirror in the men's room of some fashionable disco at 3 a.m. and thinking: "My God, did I spend all the money I spent tonight just so I could look like this?" Even then, there was no way to conceal the debilitating toll that a long, hard night of partying could take on my appearance.

Eight years ago, in 1987, I quit drinking. I weighed all the pros and cons involved, and then I made a practical, calculated decision to stop doing something that had been an ingrained part of my lifestyle for close to 35 years. Drinking was something I truly enjoyed for most of those years, at least part of the time. But at that point in my life – my mid-50s – I came to a reluctant conclusion. It was simply exacting too high a price for me to continue.

For a number of years during my 40s and early 50s, I'd been increasingly disturbed by the effect alcohol was having on my libido and sexual performance. If I had several stout drinks during the course of an evening, I noticed I not only lost interest in sex, but also lost the physical ability to do anything about it if I had been interested. As a younger guy, in my 20s and 30s, I could drink all evening and never be affected this way. But now booze was making me temporarily impotent, and that was a matter of great concern to me.

As I've repeatedly emphasized, sex is an important aspect of my life. I also happen to be convinced that an active sex life is a powerful deterrent to aging. The last thing I wanted to do was sacrifice the pleasure and health benefits of sex for a few ounces of whiskey.

To make sure it was the booze that was causing the problem, I tested myself. On nights when I would abstain from drinking completely or strictly limit myself to sipping a single cocktail, my sexual desire and performance would be unaffected. But if I drank the usual amount, the effects were obvious and undeniable.

Up until that time, I'd had no idea how commonplace this problem is and how many male drinkers experience it. It has to do with the fact that, while many people think of alcohol as a stimulant, it's actually a powerful depressant. It depresses your inhibitions, but it also depresses all your physical and mental functions. It seems to rev up your engine at first, but after a while, it throws you into a dead stall – especially if you continue to drink. That's why drunks tend to be the "life of the party" one minute and out cold the next.

Well, I decided if I had to choose between drinking and a normal sex life, there was really only one choice. I stopped drinking. I haven't had a drink since, and I never intend to start drinking again. In fact, now that I've been a non-drinker for so long, I frankly wonder why I ever started in the first place. I thought I'd miss it a lot, but I actually haven't.

Assessing a Bad Habit

Meanwhile, I've been able to make some objective assessments about drinking, based both on my many years as an active drinker and my eight years as an ex-drinker.

Except for an occasional morning-after headache and/or upset stomach, most drinkers in their 20s and 30s don't feel any serious ill-effects from their drinking. At that age, we tend to think of each separate hangover as an isolated incident unrelated to any of the others. But as it is with such other potentially destructive habits as overeating and smoking, a pattern eventually forms. There's a cumulative effect that becomes increasingly apparent after you turn 40. For overeaters, it's unwanted inches and pounds. For smokers, it's shortness of breath and a hacking cough. For drinkers, the consequences are every bit as dangerous but often much less obvious.

From time to time in our lives, most of us have encountered a few "classic" alcoholics. I'm talking about people who are simply unable to exercise any control whatsoever over their drinking. These are people who never stop drinking until they black out. People who go on binges that may last several days. People who can't hold a job or sustain a personal relationship because of their drinking. People who pose a real danger to themselves and others whenever they drink. People who seem to have to hit rock-bottom before they can come to grips with their addiction. Sometimes, they don't, even then. Sometimes, they die.

Symptoms of Dependency

But for every person who falls into this category, there are probably a dozen or two who don't display these "classic" symptoms, but who are heavily reliant on alcohol. These are men and women who average consuming five or six or seven drinks a day for many years. They aren't necessarily alcoholics – at least by my definition – but over time they develop a dependency on alcohol. That dependency is partly chemical, partly psychological. It usually intensifies as they grow older.

They may never drink before 5 o'clock in the afternoon, then have to slam down three or four drinks before they can unwind enough to go home after work. They may abstain from drinking on Mondays and Tuesdays, but then double their usual consumption on Fridays and Saturdays. They may go for a week without a drink, but then increase their dosage over the next week or two by enough to offset what they didn't drink while they were "on the wagon." I used to go for as much as 60 days myself without drinking, just to prove I could, but I could hardly wait for the 61st day when I could start again.

Besides loss of libido, long-term drinkers may also develop a variety of other physical and psychological symptoms. For example:

– Their sleep patterns are often disrupted. They may wake up in the middle of the night after sleeping soundly for three or four hours and be unable to go back to sleep. And when they sharply curtail the amount they drink, they frequently find it hard to fall asleep in the first place.

– Some become irritable, negative and hard to get along with for no discernible reason. They find it harder and harder to suppress their hostilities, both toward friends and families and toward total strangers. If they persist in trying to bolster their mood with alcohol, they can become severely depressed.

– Millions of over-40 Americans have minor but chronic gastro-intestinal disorders relating to drinking – heartburn, gas, queasiness, periodic diarrhea. Drinking is a frequent contributor to peptic ulcers, and it invariably aggravates hemorrhoids.

– While a drink or two a day may ease tension, improve circulation and increase the level of "good" HDL cholesterol in the bloodstream, sustained heavy drinking can raise blood pressure, damage the heart muscle and contribute to congestive heart failure.

– Everyone knows that alcohol abuse causes liver disease and eventual liver failure. But over-consumption also causes severe harm to the pancreas and can produce an angonizingly painful condition known as alcoholic pancreatitis. It can damage the lungs, as well, aggravating emphysema and other respiratory disorders. And, of course, it destroys vast numbers of brain cells that can never be replaced.

Alcohol and Violence

But the greatest danger to human life caused by excessive use of alcohol isn't the development of predictable disease processes. It's the threat of violent death posed by drunks to themselves and others. Dozens of people are killed by drunk drivers every day. Many others are killed by guns and knives in domestic violence and senseless brawls triggered by alcohol.

It's true that alcohol-related violence sometimes strikes at people who "never touch a drop," as well as at alcohol abusers. But I'm convinced the odds of being caught up in it and hurt or killed by it are in direct proportion to how much and how often you drink. For instance, I refuse to travel on the roads after 5 p.m. on New Year's Eve because I know how dangerous it is out there.

According to many medical experts, cigarette smoking is the number- one preventable cause of death in the world. I have no argument with that. Every year, cigarettes do kill off millions of people before their time. We have overwhelming proof that smoking causes heart attacks, strokes, lung cancer and emphysema. But if you add up all the deaths from all the various alcohol-related causes, I suspect booze runs a close second to smoking as a killer.

A Question of Limits

Anyway, these are all reasons why I'm glad I quit drinking and why I frankly wish I'd quit long before I did.

Am I advising you to quit, too? Not necessarily. But if living a long, full, productive, high-quality life ranks high on your list of priorities, I'm suggesting you at least think about it.

As you do, try to make an honest evaluation of your own personal situation. Can you really limit yourself to two (or even three) drinks a day at the max? Can you do it not just for today and tomorrow or the rest of this week or this month, but from now on? (The definition of "drink" here, by the way, is not five shots of booze with a splash of soda in a 16-ounce glass; it's the equivalent of one ounce of 90-proof liquor per drink, or about what comes in 12 ounces of beer or 5 ounces of wine. And the rules don't allow "saving up" drinks you don't have on Wednesday and Thursday in order to get totally wasted on Saturday night. The rules are no more than two or three drinks on any given day. These are the guidelines set forth by the U.S.

Surgeon General, the American Heart Association and other health authorities.)

If you can honestly answer "yes" to these questions, then go right ahead and enjoy your beer, wine or cocktails and don't worry about it. There's no medical or moral reason for you to feel guilty about drinking. There's no reason to quit drinking, either, although you probably wouldn't have any problem doing so if you decided to.

On the other hand, the unfortunate but inescapable truth is that most drinkers can't – or won't – stop at two or three drinks a day. Despite all the noble intentions in the world, those same two or three drinks will lower the inhibitions and numb the common sense of the average drinker just enough to keep him from caring at that point if he has a fourth or fifth or sixth drink or not. This is simply the nature of the beast. That's why it's actually harder for many regular "social drinkers" to drink in strict moderation than not to drink at all.

If your own experience has repeatedly borne out this fact over a long period of time, what's the point in kidding yourself? If you can't enforce two-or-three-drink-a-day limitations with no exceptions – and especially if you've spotted any of the symptoms listed above in yourself – you're better off kicking the habit entirely.

Which brings us to some other, very crucial questions: Just how hard is it to quit? How difficult is it to say, "That's it; I'm through; I'm never going to drink anymore," and then live with that decision? Can you hope to do this all by yourself, or will you have to have outside help – possibly including medical and psychological intervention?

Trying It "Cold Turkey"

There's no one pat answer to these questions. Every person is different, and a lot depends on you as an individual. But based on my own personal experiences and observations, as well as opinions I've solicited from various experts, I can offer some generalizations:

Virtually all classic alcoholics require massive doses of outside help to overcome their addiction and maintain lasting sobriety. Organizations such as Alcoholics Anonymous can sometimes pull them through the crisis. But their minds and bodies are usually so poisoned by the toxic effects of alcohol that they also have to have medical treatment, often followed up by professional counselling. Then and only then can their friends, families and AA-style groups provide the support system they need to stay sober and rebuild their lives. Recovery from classic alcoholism is usually a lifelong job.

But the same thing doesn't necessarily apply to everybody who consumes large quantities of alcohol regularly for a long period of time. Somehow, an idea has taken root in our national consciousness that says no habitual heavy drinker can quit anymore on his or her own authority or volition, that only a rigid institutionalized program under the constant monitoring of medical professionals can turn the trick. This idea isn't only false; it's utterly ridiculous. I proved this to myself eight years ago, and I know many other people who have had similar individual success.

The trouble is, today's society is permeated with a negative, defeatist philosophy when it comes to just about any kind of self-help project. We're told over and over again by the so-called "experts" that we're powerless to alter our own course or turn over a new leaf. If we want to quit smoking, we have to have a nicotine patch or be hynotized or join some organized smoking-cessation program. If we want to quit drinking, we have to check into a substance-abuse clinic to dry out. And I'm afraid this philosophy is causing a lot of people who might otherwise be able to quit smoking or drinking or drugging or whatever to give up before they even start.

The idea seems to be that none of us is responsible anymore for our own actions, that someone else is to blame for all our flaws and failings, and that, as a result, the only way to change our behavior patterns is to admit our total helplessness and turn our problem over to someone wiser and more capable.

This is pure BS as far as I'm concerned. Sure, we all need moral support from those close to us when we set out to shake a bad habit. But for every person who can't make it without costly institutional intervention, there are at least a dozen who could if they tried.

In spite of all the new and "enlightened" approaches that have been tried, the old "cold turkey" approach remains by far the most successful way to beat the cigarette habit. And smoking is a much more addictive habit than drinking. The typical smoker lights up at regular intervals 30 or 40 or 50 times a day, from the time he wakes up in the morning until he falls asleep at night. If this guy can quit cold turkey, so can the guy who's fallen into the habit of popping and drinking six or eight beers in the course of an evening.

Motivation Works Wonders

The key word is motivation. With it, you can do anything you set your mind to do. Without it, all the fancy clinics and medically approved "crutches" in the world won't keep you from taking your destructive habits to the grave with you.

One guy I know routinely downed at least a couple of drinks with his lunch every noontime for about 12 years. He said he usually came back to the office feeling pretty bouncy, but within an hour or so, his high faded. Then he started feeling muddleheaded and lethargic. It was impossible to concentrate.

"Damn it," he told me disgustedly one day, "I'm sick of feeling this way in the afternoons, and I'm not going to be a lunch-hour lush anymore. As of right now, I'm swearing off alcohol in the middle of the day."

I'm sure at least a million similar comments are made somewhere in this country every week. But the strange thing was, this acquaintance of mine really meant it. It's been more than 20 years since he told me that, and to my knowledge, he's never had a single drink at lunch in all that time.

His reasoning and motivation were ultra-simple. He didn't like what he was doing, so he didn't do it anymore. For a while, he avoided going to restaurants where alcohol was served. Instead, he would grab a sandwich at a snackbar or bring a sack lunch from home and walk down to a park near his office to eat.

When I decided to quit drinking, I remembered this man's experience and used it as a sort of example for myself. I started working out in the evenings, at a time I formerly spent with a drink in my hand. It gave me a healthy activity to substitute for an unhealthy one, just as he had substituted a walk in the park for a two-martini lunch.

Small steps like this can do a lot to break destructive patterns and keep you from slipping back into the same old rut.

Once I made up my mind about booze, I took yet another valuable cue from this same acquaintance. Just as he had told me straight out of his intention not to imbibe during the noon hour, I purposely announced my decision to anybody who would listen. The prospect of looking stupid if I reneged on the decision was just added motivation for me to go through with it.

It's a Natural Feeling

Anytime you stop doing something that's been a part of your standard routine for a long time, you're almost certain to feel a temporary sense of loss and dislocation – like something's missing. Tens of millions of people have experienced similar feelings when they quit smoking. To a large extent, it's the same way with drinking. This is only natural, and there's nothing weird or menacing about it.

Part of what you're dealing with is your body telling you you're not giving it something it's used to – in this case, alcohol. Over a period of weeks and months and years, you've administered regular doses of a chemical to yourself. Now you've cut off the supply, and your body senses the chemical's absence.

Like the craving for nicotine in an ex-smoker, this sensation will gradually decline as the days pass. But unlike the nicotine craving, which former smokers tell me can remain nearly constant for days, I think you'll find the desire for a drink tends to ebb and flow in peaks and valleys. If you're used to drinking in the early evenings – as most drinkers are – the desire will likely be at its most intense around 5:30 or 6 p.m. Oddly enough, though, you may well find it suddenly diminish around 7 or 7:30, at about the same time the traditional cocktail hour ends.

Part of the craving, of course, isn't even related to chemical dependency. Instead, it's purely pschological. The day's work is done, your subconscious tells you, and that means it's time for a drink. If you prepare yourself ahead of time to deal with these periods of peaking desire for alcohol, you'll be able to get past them with greater ease and less tension.

Easing the Transition

If and when you make the decision to quit drinking, I certainly don't advise continuing to go to the same old bar with the same old crowd each day after work. Eventually, you may be able to do this with no problem. But in the early stages of quitting, the combination of chemical and psychological need, along with peer pressure and a "boozer-friendly" atmosphere may make it impossible to sit there and sip your club soda or tonic water while everybody else ties into the hard stuff.

For the time being, the thing to do is find something else to fill the void and ease the transition. Don't let yourself be "hemmed in." Explore new territory. Broaden your horizons. Pick a location and activity that isn't associated in your mind with drinking and plunge into it. Go to a gym. Go biking or rollerblading. Go to a movie. Go swimming. Go shopping. Go to the library. Go watch your son play soccer (Hey, he's been after you for months to come to his games, anyway!).

Whatever you do, be assured that each passing day will bring you new satisfaction with your progress – and new resolve to continue. You don't have to tell yourself, "I'm never going to drink again." All you have to say is, "I'm not going to drink today." If you take care of today, tomorrow will take care of itself.

To some people, the physical act of drinking liquid is important in itself. If you've been downing a half-dozen or more alcoholic drinks every day, starving your body for liquid could aggravate its craving for alcohol. So drink plenty of water, soft drinks, iced tea, coffee, fruit juice, whatever. As long as it's non-alcoholic, who cares?

If you've been a big beer drinker, you may want to try some of the many new brands of non-alcoholic brew that have been introduced in the past two or three years. All the major national brewers and several smaller companies have their own entries in the alcohol-less beer market these days – O'Doul's from Anheuser-Busch, Cutter from Coors, Old Milwaukee NA from Stroh's, to name a few.

You may be pleasantly surprised at the drinkability of these products. They bear no resemblance to the tasteless "near-beer" of past generations, but are genuine beers, brewed in the usual way, but with all but a trace of the alcohol removed. (Legally, a non-alcoholic beverage can contain no more than 0.5 percent alcohol by volume.)

One of the best features of these brews is their low calorie content. On average, a 12-ounce bottle or can of non-alcoholic beer contains only 65 calories – or about half the number in the same amount of light beer and just over one-third the number in a regular 12-ounce beer or soft drink.

Several kinds of de-alcoholized wines and champagne are also available. It's very possible that these products can make your transition from drinker to non-drinker more comfortable.

They represent one more small reason why quitting may be easier than you think.

I want to stress one thing above all else: You have the power to do whatever you genuinely want to do where drinking, smoking and recreational drugs are concerned. If a second 50 years of healthy, fulfilling life is your goal, you also have all the motivation you need to overcome any destructive habit.

Whatever your decision may be, it's up to you. Good luck!

*"Water, taken in moderation,
cannot hurt anybody."*
–Mark Twain

CHAPTER

12

The Shocking Truth About the Water You Drink

When you turn on a faucet in your kitchen or bathroom, you probably pay little attention to the stream of crystal-clear liquid that comes gushing forth. You can leave the faucet open for as long as you want and that stream will always look the same -- sparkling, cool, refreshing.

This endless supply of fresh water is one of the marvels of the modern household. It's a convenience the kings of old couldn't buy with all their power and wealth. Just a century ago, it was a luxury that only the super-rich could afford.

Yet this water that appears so magically at the flick of a wrist is something most Americans take totally for granted. Today, at least 98 percent of all U.S. homes have it. Even those who can still remember childhood days of having to haul water in buckets from an outdoor well or pump for every household use have grown so used to "indoor plumbing" that they rarely give it a second thought anymore. Most of us never really stop to think about where the tapwater we use actually comes from.

But we should. We most definitely should. Because as pristine-pure as it looks, the water from our faucets may be dangerously contaminated with disease-producing organisms and cancer-causing chemical agents.

In fact, unknown to most of the tens of millions of Americans who drink tapwater every day, many of our public water supplies pose a severe and steadily increasing threat to public health.

"But wait a minute," you say. "The running water in my house comes through a network of pipes and mains laid by the city. It's pumped out of a government-financed reservoir, scientifically treated at a municipal water plant, tested regularly for impurities, and certified to be safe for human consumption."

Overcoming Ignorance

All this is true, of course. Water for public use is managed and monitored and treated and certified. Things have changed drastically since most folks got their drinking water from shallow, hand-dug wells or flowing streams or natural springs. Back in those days, there were few laws or standards governing drinking water. Sometimes, water was clean enough, simply because there weren't that many people around to get it dirty. Other times, it could be deadly.

The homesteader who casually dipped up a bucket of water from a gurgling little creek was often oblivious to the cow pastures, hogpens and outhouses whose byproducts flowed into it upstream. There was a widely held belief that as long as water flowed over rocks for some distance, it was OK to drink. In cities and towns, noxious commercial wastes frequently leached into unlined wells. Mainly as a result of ignorance and primitive conditions, Americans contracted many dread diseases from their water.

When science discovered that microbes were to blame for these diseases and that many of them flourished in water, modern water treatment technology began to develop, and public water supplies became safer than they had ever been before.

But as our population has soared and we've found more and more sophisticated ways to fill our water with poisons, this technology hasn't been able to keep pace. The result is a new surge in water-related disease.

"But this is the U.S.A – not some third-world country," you protest. "We have the highest sanitary standards of any nation on earth. How can the water I use every day be a threat to anybody's health?"

The explanation for how our water got in its current dangerous condition is long and involved. At the moment, it's a problem without a solution. And until our federal, state and local governments find and enforce that solution – if they ever do – it's up to us as individuals to take whatever steps may be necessary to protect ourselves.

Some Stunning Statistics

Listen to the shocking findings of a recent study carried out by two major environmental organizations, using data compiled by the federal Environmental Protection Agency and local water utilities across the country:

– More than 53 million Americans are drinking tapwater contaminated by lead, fecal bacteria, toxic chemicals and other pollutants.

– More than 7 million cases of mild to moderate illness are caused each year by contaminated water.

– At least 1,200 people will be killed this year by the water they drink.

When these frightening statistics were first reported in June 1995, they stunned even many experts in the field of water pollution. Some of these experts had been warning for years that the levels of contaminants in our water were steadily climbing, but most were unaware of how severe the problem has already become. The figures were far higher than earlier estimates of the impact of waterborne diseases on the general population.

My purpose here isn't to be an alarmist or cause anyone to panic. The chances of your being struck down by some sudden, dread disease the next time you drink a glass of tapwater are virtually nonexistent. Unlike the era when typhoid and other bacterial diseases ran rampant because of impure drinking water, most of the danger associated with contaminated water today is of the long-term variety.

But it's my belief that water pollution has reached such proportions in this country that it has to be considered an important factor affecting the overall health and longevity of Americans everywhere. Even worse, the problem appears to be out of control, with no real solution in sight. This indicates to me that the situation is likely to get worse over the next few years before effective counter-measures can be taken to reduce the risk.

That's why I've taken concrete steps to protect myself. After you read this chapter, there's a good chance you may want to do the same.

Undoubtedly, there are still many localities in the U.S. where the drinking water remains clean and free of contaminants. But if 53 million Americans – roughly one-fifth of our total population – are drinking polluted water, can any of us blithely continue to assume our water is safe?

In North Texas, where I live, we don't have nearly as much industrial pollution as, say, the Northeast. But even here, the concentration of chemicals in our public water supply is far too high, and the interaction of these chemicals with the chlorine added in the treatment of raw water is creating potential perils that can only be guessed at today. It only stands to reason that the situation is far more dangerous in other more populous, more heavily industrialized parts of the country.

Technology Falls Behind

My first inkling of the amount of disease-causing organisms and toxic substances contained in our water came several years ago when I met a young water scientist named Bruce Huther.

Huther is a former pro football player for the Dallas Cowboys who stayed in the Dallas area after he retired from sports to get his graduate degree in aquatic toxicology. Later, he formed his own company, Huther & Associates, a consulting firm which helps municipal water suppliers in the area conform with clean-water standards established by the federal government.

The trouble is, though, they often can't conform.

"It's impossible to take everything potentially harmful out of the water supply," Huther says, "because the technology just isn't there – at least not yet. If we eventually develop the technology, it's going to be expensive. Even now, cities don't have the money to treat water as efficiently as it should be treated, so the question will become, 'How much are we, as taxpayers, willing to spend for pure water?'"

Basically, there are two main types of pollutants: (1) Bacteria and other disease-causing micro-organisms, and (2) chemical toxins ranging from the pesticides and insecticides used in farming to the waste compounds discharged in industrial manufacturing to the heavy metals released by electrical generating plants.

Traditionally, chlorine has been added to water to kill whatever harmful bacteria it may contain. But adding chlorine does nothing to remove or neutralize the various chemical toxins that may remain in the water indefinitely, even after repeated filterings. On the contrary, the chlorine can interact with the chemicals to produce compounds known as trihalomethanes, which are known carcinogens.

Compounding the Problem

Many people are deeply concerned today over the fact that treated wastewater, or effluent, is now routinely discharged into water-supply reservoirs just a short distance from the intakes where drinking water is being pumped from the same reservoir. I can understand their concern.

This is a standard procedure in the Dallas/Fort Worth Metroplex and many other major metropolitan areas. Only in mountainous regions where most drinking water is derived from melting snow and man-made reservoirs aren't widely used is it less common.

To me, the knowledge that this is being done more and more frequently is unnerving if not downright nauseating. The utilities, however, maintain that this "pipe-to-pipe" situation is perfectly harmless, because the treated effluent from modern wastewater plants (they don't call them "sewer plants" anymore) is subject to such stringent federal regulations. And in populous urban areas, it makes little sense to try to keep wastewater and whatever pollutants it contains away from public drinking-water supplies within the same watershed. Sooner or later, it's all going to end up in the same place, anyway.

Ironically, it is true that treated effluent is required to be purer at the time it's discharged into reservoirs than the actual drinking water that flows through our faucets – at least where the level of trihalomethanes is concerned. The tiny aquatic organisms placed in the treated effluent to test its purity can live in it with no problem. But when chlorine is added to kill whatever bacteria remain in the water, it also makes the water lethal to the test organisms. Meanwhile, minuscule residues of chemical contaminants remain to mix with the chlorine, producing trihalomethanes and potentially bigger problems.

"Our wastewater treatment plants are constructed to treat and remove sewage from water, not to get rid of chemical contaminants," Huther explains. "So a residue of these chemicals remains in treated wastewater, and the residue becomes more dangerous to health when chlorine is added to the water. On a long-term basis, the chemical hazard we face today is more dangerous than the bacteria the chlorine is intended to destroy."

Some Toxins Last Forever

Scientists are looking for alternative means of purification, especially sophisticated new systems of filtration for removing chemicals, but this is a painfully slow process. Meanwhile, some of the toxic materials entering our water supply may be impossible to remove later.

"The big companies are cranking out new kinds of chemicals all the time, for which no effective treatment is available," Huther says, "and some pesticides don't biodegrade, or break down, with the passage of time. Some of them just stick around forever. At the moment, the only thing the utilities know to do is hit the water with larger doses of chlorine, and this may only aggravate the problem."

Some of the worst corporate polluters try to dodge the law by discharging carcinogenic chemicals secretly. Often it takes a year or two from the time a toxicity problem is found for investigators to pinpoint a particular source of chemical pollution. Then the offender is automatically allowed a three-year period of variance by the EPA, during which it can continue to pollute. And so the problem grows.

To complicate matters still further, not all the disease-causing micro-organisms at which it is aimed are killed by chlorinization. Some have developed a high level of resistence.

"The hepatitis virus, for example, can pass right through a treatment plant without being fazed," Huther points out.

A Real-Life Outbreak?

This is all scary stuff. It scares me, and I don't mind admitting it. The news is full of horror stories about new strains of viruses that are immune to any weapon medical science can throw at them. What if one of these strains got loose in the public water supply of a major U.S. city? As farfetched as it may seem, we could witness a catastrophe similar to the one portrayed in Dustin Hoffman's recent movie *Outbreak*.

I don't like to think about things like that, but sometimes I can't help myself.

Up until a few years ago, though, I was just as unconcerned as the next person about the water that flowed from the faucets in my house. My real concern started after my first lengthy conversation with Bruce, who had served a stint as an inspector for the City of Dallas Water Department before forming his own consulting firm.

One of Bruce's jobs was to check on what type of pollutants various businesses and institutions were dumping down their drains and into the municipal sewer system. What he found was shocking, even to a toxicologist. Funeral homes were flushing embalming fluid and the wastes from cadavers directly into the sanitary sewer system. Hospitals were doing the same with the wastes from thousands of patients suffering from infectious diseases ranging from AIDS to hepatitis to influenza.

"All I could do was give the worst offenders a citation and try to persuade the others to take greater precautions," he says. "I'm not sure how much good either approach did."

So what can we do as individuals to minimize the hidden hazards that may be concealed in our innocent-looking tapwater?

Steps for Self-Protection

Obviously, most of us can't totally avoid using water from a public water supply. But there are steps we can take – some easy and inexpensive, some more costly and complex – to minimize the risk to our health.

For instance, instead of filling your glass immediately when the water's been turned off overnight or longer, let the tap run for a minute or so first. Evaporation can cause water left standing in pipes for hours or days to develop a high concentration of heavy metals. Under these circumstances, water can also lose its chlorinization, allowing bacteria to form.

It also doesn't cost much, either in money or inconvenience, to add bottled water to your supermarket shopping list and keep a jug of it in the refrigerator for drinking. Remember, though, only distilled bottled water is free of chemical additives and impurities. Bottled spring water, like tapwater, is usually chlorinated.

Five gallons of bottled water a week will usually take care of two people's personal needs for drinking water, making coffee or tea, mixing frozen juices, etc.

If you want to spend $200 to $500, you can install a charcoal filter on the cold water intake under your kitchen sink that will remove many contaminants and also absorb the chlorine in your tapwater. If you take this route, it's vitally important to be sure to change the filter cartridges often. One $30 cartridge lasts about three months on average, but if you keep using the filter after it gets dirty, you may end up with worse contamination than if you had no filter at all.

My own personal solution – and one that's given me considerable peace of mind since I had it done – was to install a distillation system in my house that provides plenty of running distilled water for drinking, cooking and other kitchen uses. The system cost $2,500, which may be more than most people would be willing to pay, but to me, it's been worth every penny.

For one thing, it eliminates the need to lug heavy jugs of water around – something I still do on my frequent trips to Mexico, where sanitation and water purification are still primitive in comparison to the U.S.

Clare and I even give our pets distilled water and use it for our house plants. The difference in the way those plants look since we started them on a distilled-water "diet" is enough in itself to convince me it must also be good for people.

We still use tapwater for bathing, showering, shampooing and other household uses. And when I go to a restaurant or someone else's home or office where the water isn't distilled, I don't worry about it. As I said, it's the long-term, day-after-day exposure to most pollutants that pose the greatest danger. An occasional swallow of tapwater isn't likely to cause any serious harm.

We're All Responsible

All of us need to be aware of the enormity of our water pollution problem. You may not read nearly as much about it, but it's every bit as big a threat to our health and well-being as air pollution or food contamination. We need to support governmental efforts to stop industrial polluters and severely penalize those who violate the law. At the same time, though, we also need to realize that millions of us ordinary citizens unwittingly play a small part in water pollution.

When was the last time you painted with a water-base paint, then washed out your brush and roller in the sink? Have you ever cleaned silver, copper or brass with a strong, caustic solution and let the residue run down the drain? How often have you flushed a chemical cleaner, leftover cosmetics, or some kind of solvent down the commode? How much weedkiller, insecticide and chemical fertilizer gets sprayed on your lawn each spring?

These and many other seemingly harmless acts contribute significantly to our water pollution crisis, especially when they happen millions of times each year.

While we need to take immediate steps to protect our own health and safety, we should also be thinking about the health and safety of future generations. Unless we do, the crisis is only going to get worse.

"Love makes time pass, and time makes love pass."
–AMERICAN PROVERB

CHAPTER 13

Maintaining a Healthy, Active Sex Life to 100 or Beyond

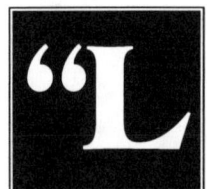

"**L**ove makes the world go 'round," as the old saying goes. And although there are many other aspects of romantic love, sexual arousal and fulfillment have always been – and always will be – the "engine" that powers it.

Can you remember your first serious romance? The first time you engaged in the ultimate acts of intimacy with someone you really cared deeply about? The first time you really made love?

I'm not necessarily talking just about your first sexual encounter. That might have been something entirely different – a mere physical experience, and not necessarily even a pleasant one, at that. Your first brush with sex might have been an accident of fate or a fleeting one-night stand with a partner you never saw again. That isn't what I mean.

What I'm referring to is the first time you ever actually felt the full, electrifying impact of loving and being loved.

Remember the boost to your ego and emotions? Remember the indescribable feeling of exhilaration, the sense of giving and receiving mutual satisfaction? Remember feeling like you were 10 feet tall and had the world by the tail?

If you can't remember, better have your memory checked right away. There's no greater high than the one you get through the magical sensations of first love. But sexuality isn't meant to end with first love – or second or third or fourth love, for that matter. Whether you remain with one mate or share love with dozens of partners, that high is something worth striving to repeat an infinite number of times throughout your life.

In a biological sense, our main purpose on this earth is to procreate, to reproduce, to carry on our species. Without sex, this is impossible. Therefore, a life devoid of sexual attraction, sexual stimulation and sexual activity is a life from which a giant share of meaning and purpose has been stolen.

So what happens when the "engine" breaks down or runs out of gas? At this point, I believe a profound change begins to take place in an individual. The aging process accelerates. An ominous pattern takes shape. Something inside a person begins to die.

That's why I intend to maintain a healthy, active sex life for as long as I live. I don't think there has to be a cutoff point for romance and sexual fulfillment. In one of the most famous stories of the Old Testament, God gave Abraham the power to father a son, and his wife, Sarah, the ability to bear that son when they both were in their 90s. This phenomenon may never be repeated in our time, since few people would choose to have a child at such an advanced age, even if it were physically possible. But modern science is enabling us to maintain the sexual feelings and functions that would make such a miracle possible longer than ever before.

A Man's Special Problem

What about you? How long has it been since sex was a major, motivating part of your life? What status does it have with you today? Is it something you simply try not to think about? Something that exists mostly in the dark corners of your memory? Something you may even shy away from for fear of disappointing your partner and/or embarrassing yourself?

If any of these descriptions pop into your mind, I want you to understand one basic fact: It doesn't have to be that way!

For obvious anatomical reasons, males have a much more

pronounced problem than females when their sex drive diminishes. Even when a women is indifferent or downright bored, she can always "fake it" or be a passive participant in the sex act. But unless a man is sexually aroused enough to maintain an erection, he simply can't perform. Rare is the man past 40 who hasn't at least occasionally encountered a situation where "the spirit is willing, but the flesh is weak."

After 40, many factors can cause or contribute to male sexual dysfunction and impotence. I've already mentioned such factors as drinking too much alcohol, chronic depression, prostate problems and the side effects of certain prescription medications.

Many of us think of the loss of sex drive as a purely physical failing. As one friend of mine asks disgustedly: "Why is it so easy to get stiff everywhere except the one part of my body that really matters?"

The Mechanics of Erection

Maybe the best way to start answering that question is to explain the two basic physiological processes that produce and maintain an erection.

First, enough blood must flow into the penis via the cavernosus artery to fill a network of expandable sacs in the organ. The inflowing blood inflates these sacs like thousands of tiny balloons and makes the penis rigid. Simultaneously, the veins that normally drain blood out of these sacs constrict, trapping the blood in the penis and keeping it from flowing back out.

Recent studies show that, under normal conditions, the inflow of blood begins when stimulation causes the nerve endings in the penis to release nitric oxide, which, in turn, relaxes smooth muscle tissue and lets the blood enter the sacs.

When there is insufficient blood flow to the penis in the first place, the erection is either only partial or completely non-existent. And when the blood is released too quickly back into the veins, whatever erection is obtained is lost before it can serve its purpose.

Obviously, anything that impedes blood flow is likely to decrease the ability to produce an erection – whether it's hardening of the arteries or a simple lack of stimulation to the nerve ends so that not enough nitric oxide is released. And conditions such as "venous leakage," which allow blood to seep out of the penis, can make an erection impossible to retain for a sufficient length of time.

What Every Woman Needs

While a woman doesn't have to maintain an erection to have sex, this doesn't mean that she's immune to physical problems related to advancing age. These problems frequently make sexual activity difficult if not impossible and rob her of even the slightest pleasure.

After menopause, the vagina tends to become narrower, shorter, dryer and less elastic. Even worse, its walls become thinner and subject to injury and/or infection.

Compounding the problem is the fact that a woman's libido also tends to dry up, in part probably because of the pain involved in sex. In effect, both the physical and psychological centers of sexual activity simply shut down, and unless something is done, they may remain that way for life.

None of this has to happen, however. There's usually a simple but miraculous cure for this whole unhappy condition. It's called estrogen.

Estrogen replacement therapy (ERT) can relieve all these symptoms almost overnight. Estrogen creams or gels can rejuvenate the vaginal tissues and restore natural lubrication, and a daily estrogen tablet can reawaken a woman's sexuality and keep it awake for decades. Some gynecologists use estrogen injections to keep a woman's libido fine-tuned. If a woman in her 40s or 50s loses interest in sex, a simple test can determine whether her estrogen is lower than it should be, and monthly injections can quickly raise it to the desired level – that of a 20-year-old. To give the libido an added boost, testosterone can be injected along with the estrogen. Each woman can decide for herself how much of an increase in libido she wants and have her doctor adjust the hormone dosages accordingly.

"Even for women who are already in deep sexual difficulty, the (estrogen) therapy usually reverses the damage in only a few weeks," says Dr. Lila Nachtigall, co-author of *Estrogen: The Facts Can Change Your Life*, in a recent *Time* article.

As mentioned in an earlier chapter, ERT offers important health and anti-aging benefits both before and after menopause. And for any woman in her 40s, 50s or 60s, it can also mean a new lease on your sex life.

"Without it," says Dr. Nachtigall, "you may soon have no sex life at all."

When the Thrill Is Gone

In addition to physical factors, there are many psychological causes for a lagging libido and male impotency problems. Personal or job-related stresses and pressures, for example, can be a major villain. So can the deadening effects of a stagnant relationship.

For one reason or another, those initial romantic thrills seem to grow more and more difficult to duplicate as the years roll by. After 20 or 30 or 40 years of marriage, there's often little romance left between husbands and wives. In many cases, it isn't that they've quit caring about each other; it's just that the distractions of everyday life and the same old routine effectively stifle their sexual impulses. Men stop saying and doing the "little things" that trigger a romantic response in their mates. Women, for their part, find it too much trouble to look attractive or behave seductively toward their spouses.

Frequently, the prolonged absence of romance and intimacy leads to separation and divorce. Some people's efforts to recapture it become a compulsive thing that keeps them continually switching mates or partners. Some prowl the nightclubs, bars and dancehalls in search of "Mr. or Ms. Right." But the results seldom live up to their hopes or expectations.

For one reason or another, by the time most men and women are in their 50s and 60s, they've convinced themselves that the wonderful, stimulating high of sex at its best has been forever left behind in the past. The "engine" seems to have developed burned-out bearings and a flat crankshaft. It looks as if the next stop is the junkyard.

"Oh, well," millions of people tell themselves, "losing interest in sex is just part of getting older."

I say, "Come on, get real! Stop deluding yourself." The fact is, there are steps anyone can take to disprove this self-defeating idea.

When Men Try Too Hard

The first thing both men and women need to understand is that when no identifiable physical cause can be found for a male's inability to perform, it's usually only a temporary condition. Sometimes, as I've said, it happens because his wife or lover no longer appeals to him in a romantic way. On the other hand, it can frequently happen when a woman is too attractive to the man pursuing her. He may try too hard and worry too much about pleasing her. Then, when the big moment arrives, he's such a nervous wreck that he can't do anything about it.

"Every male will have an experience where he knows circumstances are right for an erection, but it just doesn't happen," says Dr. Jay B. Hollander, associate director of the Beaumont Center for Male Sexual Function in Royal Oak, Michigan. "That can really scare a person. It shouldn't, because it's usually a temporary phenomenon. But the more you worry about it, the more it gets into your brain, which increases your chances of dysfunction the next time."

One "cure" for this problem is simply not to try so hard. Ironically, the smooth muscles of the penis have to relax to allow the inflow of blood that produces an erection. If every other muscle in your body is tense with anxious expectation, it's only natural to assume that these muscles are tense, too.

It's also important not to rush sex. Far from being a chore to hurry through, the "love play" or foreplay that prepares you and your mate for sexual fulfillment should be just as pleasureable as the act itself. And getting ready may take longer than it used to. There are lots of things you don't expect to be able to do as fast at 50 or 60 as you do at 20 or 30, and a man's penis may not respond to stimulation as quickly, either. Allow plenty of time to reach a state of full arousal.

A man may also need more time to "recharge his batteries" between episodes of lovemaking. Even if he was the kind of guy at 25 who thought no day (or night) was complete without sex, he may very well find at 50 that once or twice a week – or even less often – is plenty. The frequency with which you have sex is less important than the quality of the experience when you do have it.

If problems persist and a medical exam reveals no physical cause for impotence, psychological counseling can often help. For help in finding a qualified counselor, call the American Association of Sex Educators, Counselors and Therapists at (312) 644-0828 or the Impotence Institute of America at (800) 669-1603.

Tracing Physical Causes

Remember, too, that you aren't alone in this. The landmark Massachusetts Male Aging Study showed that well over half of all men between the ages of 40 and 70 have regular and recurring impotency problems. At 40, the percentage is about one-third, and it climbs to two-thirds among 70-year-olds. Presumably, the problems are even more prevalent in older men, but few studies have been done on that age group, probably on the assumption that sex is virtually non-existent among males in their 70s, 80s and 90s.

The Massachusetts study and others suggest a strong correlation between impotence and certain physical disorders associated with advancing age. It is known, for example, that diabetes causes nerve damage which increases the odds of impotence. Men with high blood pressure and heart disease are also more likely to become impotent. If untreated, peptic ulcers, arthritis and some allergies can cause total impotence. A high level of "good" HDL cholesterol in the bloodstream seems to decrease the chances of impotence, possibly because it keeps the blood circulating more freely through the arteries.

Smokers are especially likely to develop impotence – about three times as likely as heart disease patients who don't smoke, according to research findings. And, surprisingly, impotence strikes more active, athletic males than it does couch potatoes, simply because the former suffer more sports-related injuries to the crotch area. By some estimates, 600,000 American men are affected sexually by injuries that impair blood flow to the groin.

If you have a problem with sexual dysfunction that could be traced to one of these physical causes, you'd obviously be wise to see your doctor and check out some of medicine's amazing new approaches to overcome impotence.

No More "Hopeless Cases"

Scientific research is taking giant strides in this field. Eventually, I believe impotence will be wiped out completely for anyone willing to take advantage of available treatments. Dr. Ken Goldberg, a urologist who heads the Male Health Center in Dallas, sums up the confidence of today's medical profession when he says: "We can get any man an erection in the 1990s."

This is no exaggeration. Recently developed drugs called vasodilators can cause erections even in patients with spinal cord damage. A single injection of one of these drugs into the penis produces an erection within a few minutes that lasts up to three hours. I have a close friend in his mid-70s who has used vasodilators any number of times with no problems and complete satisfaction (no pun intended).

The idea of piercing your penis with a needle sounds painful, I know. But the small-gauge insulin needle used to inject the drug minimizes any discomfort, and people like my friend report near-miraculous results. Some men find their potency increases even after they stop the injections, and doctors think the drugs may produce long-term improvements in blood flow in the artery that supplies the penis.

I can tell you right now that I'd have no hesitation about using this type of drug myself if circumstances warranted. It means that a physically active man of 80 or 90 can satisfy a woman of any age.

The vasodilators work by mimicking the body's natural "triggers" for an erection, and research is moving forward on other medications that may be even more effective and not require an injection.

In addition, there are vacuum pumps available for about $400 that produce an erection by creating negative pressure around the penis and allowing blood to flow in. The user then places an elastic ring around the base of the penis to keep the blood from flowing out.

Penile implants are a last resort, which I don't necessarily recommend, because I believe there are other answers that are more practical, less expensive and every bit as effective. Implants are irreversible, since the procedure destroys the spongy tissue inside the penis. But the latest implant devices are much more sophisticated than earlier versions, which were nothing more than rigid, bendable wires. Today's hydraulic implants can be pumped up as needed.

Other, even better solutions to the impotency problem are on the horizon. Here's what a recent article in *Health & Fitness* magazine has to say on the subject:

"The sheer volume of ongoing research also augurs well for new solutions to flagging performance. Armed with fresh insights into the biochemistry of erections, researchers are developing medications and delivery systems less draconian than puncturing your organ with a hypodermic needle. For instance,

Zonagen, a Houston biotech firm, is working on an oral medicine that relaxes the smooth muscles of the penis and ideally leads to an erection within 15 minutes of taking it. In Israel, scientists have developed a topical lotion called Stearyl-VIP that may one day help men who have diseases such as diabetes anoint their way to arousal. And there could be federal approval as early as 1997 for a pill that amplifies the brain's nerve signals to the penis, thus putting a man in the mood and posture for love."

The Case for Testosterone

I've already touched briefly on the relationship between levels of testosterone, the male sex hormone, and libido, particularly in men. I've been convinced for a long time that maintaining a high testosterone level is the single most important key to a man's ability to continue a healthy, active sex life far into his second 50 years. And my own personal experience has borne this out time after time.

Testosterone can not only keep your "engine" running at full power. It can also help you combat the overall effects of aging. The typical testosterone level of a 20-year-old male is in the 800 to 1,200 range, but by the time this same man reaches his 50s, his testosterone has likely declined to the 200 range or below.

I have my testosterone checked every few months. When it gets below 400 or so, I get an injection, and I can feel the positive results. I also know that when my testosterone level dips – once it dropped down to about 140 – it touches off a negative chain reaction in my body. I gain body fat, lose lean muscle mass, and can almost feel myself aging.

While it's a male hormone, testosterone can often help boost a woman's libido, too. When a woman takes testosterone, the dosage should be carefully monitored by her doctor, however. Too much can cause an increase in body hair or other undesirable side effects.

Most doctors will administer testosterone shots only if you ask for them, but I strongly recommend that you do ask if you're experiencing sexual difficulties. I predict you'll notice a difference in both your sex drive and your general approach to life. Over a period of many years, testosterone has been shown to increase a person's energy, productivity and competitiveness. I've suspected for a long time that many political leaders and corporate CEOs have especially high testosterone levels. I also wonder if that old expression, "He's got the balls for the job," may not be more accurate than many people realize.

Incidentally, a testosterone gel is also now available. It can be applied externally to the testes. It can help to maintain an adequate level of the hormone between injections.

Another medication that has proved highly beneficial in combatting impotency is yohimbine, an extract of the bark of an African tree, available by perscription. The results of two authoritative studies show 20 to 40 percent of men can be helped by yohimbine. That's why I take three 5.4-milligram tablets of it daily.

Keeping Your Sex Appeal

The bottom line is this: Given the modern scientific knowledge at our disposal, there's absolutely no reason ever to forfeit the high of sex at any age. Even at 100 or more, you can continue to perform sexually if you want to.

Injections, implants and penile inflation may not allow you to recreate all the excitement and sensation of your earlier sexual experiences. But providing pleasure and fulfillment to your mate is also an integral part of that experience, and these techniques make it possible for you to keep right on doing this.

Beyond today's science and technology, however, it's worth remembering that "sexy is as sexy does." Sex appeal is something that comes naturally and effortlessly to only a handful of people, regardless of age. For the other 99 percent of us, it has to be cultivated and nurtured to make it blossom. Whether you're 17 or 77, putting forth a conscious effort to keep yourself attractive and appealing to the opposite sex is almost certain to pay dividends. On the other hand, don't expect your spouse to spend a lot of time and effort keeping up his or her own appearance if you're always moping around looking like something the cat dragged in.

Be positive about yourself and your significant other. Stop taking it for granted that he/she isn't interested in making love anymore or is no longer turned on by your attentions. If he/she acts uninterested, it's probably just a reflection of the way you act.

Don't sit around waiting for your mate to make the first move. If you do, you may spend the rest of your life in a stalemate.

Instead, take the initiative. Make it a point to set aside regular times and places in your life for intimacy and romance. Do something special together once in a while, but in the meantime, don't neglect to say and do the small things that promote that "just the two of us" feeling.

Remember, you're never too old to whisper those incomparable, unforgettable three little words:

"I want you!"

*"The art of medicine consists of amusing
the patient while nature cures the disease."*
–VOLTAIRE

CHAPTER

14

Beware of the "Health Hucksters"

When you adopt a healthier, more vigorous lifestyle and set your sights on living a longer, fuller, more satisfying life, you're doing yourself the greatest favor imaginable. Virtually every step you take toward that end becomes an asset and an advantage to you. Virtually every sacrifice you make is offset by a larger corresponding dividend.

But everything in this world has its down side, it seems. And if there's a negative aspect to placing a high priority on fitness and longevity, it has to be the many sophisticated con artists, charlatans and fly-by-nighters who are all too ready to sell you worthless or overpriced products and services in the name of better health and longer life.

There's no limit to the money you can waste on these "health hucksters" and their scams, but the more you're willing to spend, the more they tend to swarm around and take advantage of you. They come in all shapes and sizes, and they ballyhoo an incredibly array of products – from $1,000-a-day "longevity clinics" to slickly packaged, nationally advertised concoctions that promise health, youthfulness, pep, ideal weight and good looks for just four or five bucks a bottle

In my half-century as a devoted "health nut," I've encountered every conceivable type of gouging, false advertising, deception and out-and-out lies. I've learned how to spot and avoid the people who perpetrate these frauds, and it's my hope that I can help you steer clear of them as well.

Some of them can be ruinously expensive – not only in terms of dollars spent needlessly but in terms of time and effort wasted on programs and products that do nothing to lengthen life, benefit health or improve the way you look and feel.

Preying on Desperation

To me, there's nothing more pathetic – or more infuriating – than to see someone suffering from an incurable illness and being simultaneously victimized by purveyors of false hope. Yet patients with dread diseases are among the most frequent targets for the most unscrupulous of these vultures. Deluded by vague claims and nebulous promises of miracle cures, some desperate patients will go to any length and spend every cent they can get their hands on for worthless pills and elixirs or meaningless treatments with phony machines.

Thousands of Americans, for example, have spent staggering sums of money on so-called chelation therapy. This is an unauthorized procedure sometimes carried out by practitioners without recognized medical degrees, in which chemicals are injected into the arteries and which, proponents claim, can reverse atherosclerosis, the deadly process that blocks coronary arteries and leads to heart attacks.

No evidence exists that this treatment has ever cured anyone of coronary heart disease, but there's indisputable proof that people have died because they put their faith – and money – into chelation therapy instead of reducing the known risk factors and receiving competent conventional treatment.

Even with all the huge recent strides in combatting and slowing life-threatening disease processes after they've been diagnosed, reasonable people have to face facts: Medicine does still have its limitations. At this moment, there simply is no known cure for such diseases as atherosclerosis, cancer, diabetes, Parkinsonism and Alzheimer's.

And if all of organized medicine hasn't found a cure, what are the odds of buying one that actually works from some maverick researcher on the fringes of science? Realistically, next to none. In my opinion, anyone who tells you otherwise is most likely a crook or an idiot.

It may be intriguing to speculate about, say, a secret cancer cure lurking out there somewhere while "the establishment" connives to keep it from the public. But with today's instant global communications, I think it's basically impossible to hush up something of such magnitude. If it had legitimate value, I doubt that even the FDA could suppress the knowledge of it for very long.

Still, it's easy to understand why critically ill people often refuse to accept hard facts like these. And because of their willingness to deny the truth and try anything that might help – regardless of how far-out and bizarre – they are often easy prey for bogus "bootleg cures" and those who callously promote them.

On the other hand, it never hurts to explore all available options. My advice to anyone who feels doubtful, uncertain or suspicious of a doctor's diagnosis and/or recommended course of treatment is to get a second opinion, and maybe even a third or fourth.

A Fateful False Alarm

Remember, there are hundreds of thousands of people walking around in this world today who would have been dead and buried long ago if their ills had been accurately diagnosed and their medical prognoses had been correct.

Whenever I think of a botched diagnosis, I think of an old friend of mine named Gary. When Gary was in his early 40s, he was a heavy smoker and grossly overweight. His diet was terribly high in fat, and he never exercised. One day, he started having chest pains at work and was rushed by ambulance to a hospital.

Everyone, including the doctors, assumed – quite logically – that Gary had had a massive heart attack. He was placed in intensive care and hooked up to an oxygen tank. His family and friends were almost sure he was going to die, and so was Gary.

After about a day, test results showed that Gary hadn't had a heart attack at all. His problem was a painful but harmless spasm of the esophagus. Otherwise, he was in surprisingly good shape.

But as it turned out, Gary's false alarm was a blessing in disguise. He quit smoking, lost weight, got on an exercise program, and generally changed his whole lifestyle. Today, some 16 years later, Gary is the picture of health and vitality.

"I feel like God gave me a reprieve back there," he says, "and I made up my mind to take full advantage of it. The funny thing is, if I'd kept on like I was going, I'm sure I would've had a heart attack for real."

For the rest of us, the message here is simple: Taking the common-sense steps that anyone can take to improve his or her health is far more beneficial than spending your time, energy and money in search of nebulous miracle cures or magical shields against disease.

Fighting for Survival

"An ounce of prevention is worth a pound of cure" is much more to me than just another old saying. It's an axiom that I live by every day.

Once a major disease process has invaded your body and set up shop there, your chances of living a full, satisfying second 50 years are greatly diminished. This is the undeniable truth, and it's the chief reason why my whole approach to health and longevity is built around the concept of prevention.

But this doesn't mean that the basic tenets of building and preserving good health don't apply to someone with a serious, life-threatening illness. They definitely do. I firmly believe that proper nutrition, regular exercise, the cessation of destructive habits and a positive psychological attitude can do more than all the medications in the world to improve the quality of life and extend the survival period of someone with an incurable disease.

For some people, accepting the idea that they will never be completely "well" again in a medical sense simply means giving up. But those who want to survive intensely enough to change their lifestyle for the better often find a whole new lease on life. Frequently, they amaze their doctors. Sometimes, they even outlive them. I've seen it happen.

There was this other friend of mine, for instance. I'll call her Tina.

Tina loved to play tennis, and she was really good at the game. Unfortunately, she also liked to smoke cigarettes. Shortly after her 45th birthday, Tina developed a terrible cough that refused to go away. When she finally went for a checkup, she was diagnosed with inoperable cancer in both lungs. The doctors gave her six months – at the outside.

Tina was stunned, of course. But to her credit, the first thing she did was throw away her cigarettes. She never smoked one again.

"They say I can't play tennis anymore," she told me defiantly. "But I'm going to show them!"

Tina consulted a nutritionist and started following a nutrition program that was high in protein and complex carbohydrates and low in fat. She augmented her diet with liberal vitamin and mineral supplements. And she played tennis five or six times a week. Even during chemotherapy, she rarely missed a day going to the tennis court.

Tina and her husband were quite wealthy, incidentally. She had the means to travel anywhere and consult the finest specialists. So she could have spent all her time and money chasing around the globe in search of revolutionary new treatments, but she didn't. In doing so, she could easily have overlooked the basic elements of building up and maintaining what health she had left. But to her credit, Tina realized that would've been a poor trade.

About nine months after her cancer was diagnosed, new tests and x-rays revealed some incredible results. The cancer was still there in both of Tina's lungs, but it had stopped spreading. It was as if it had somehow been sealed off from the healthy tissue around it. Tina looked great. She said she felt great, too. And her tennis game had never been better.

Tina enjoyed a full, active life for almost eight years – or more than 15 times as long as the doctors had originally given her to live. Armed with nothing more than guts and good sense, she beat the odds. In the process, she became an inspiration to everyone who knew her, including dozens of other cancer patients.

To me, Tina's case shows that, even when it's too late to prevent disease, there's still time to reap the benefits of good nutrition, vigorous exercise, a clean lifestyle and a positive outlook.

If she had ignored these factors in favor of some ultra-expensive, ultra-far-out "cancer cure" formulated from apricot seeds, I suspect the doctors' original prognosis would have come a lot closer to being accurate.

I've always admired Tina for her courage and spirit. I only wish she'd taken better care of her health while her disease was still in the preventable stage.

Snake Oil for Suckers

Companies and individuals who advertise effortless shortcuts to health, strength and well-being in the 1990s are no different from the medicine show pitchmen of the 19th century who hawked concoctions they claimed would cure everything from tuberculosis to ingrown toenails. The approaches used today may be more modern and sophisticated, but in reality, the snake oil they are designed to sell is just as worthless as it ever was.

For example, I can't tell you how many products I've seen advertised as "fat burners" over the years. Believe me, there's simply no such thing as a nutrient or chemical that miraculously burns off fat. The only real fat burners are amphetamines, which are extremely dangerous, so don't let yourself be ripped off.

Getting rid of fat isn't an easy job. Neither is building and maintaining health. These tasks have never been easy, and they never will be. Success requires will power, discipline and motivation. These are the only indispensable components in the formula.

It's hard to break old habits. It requires perseverance to quit smoking, especially if you've been puffing a pack or two of cigarettes for 25 or 30 years. Nobody can exercise without sweating. It takes work and determination to shrink inches from your waistline. And no matter what you may read or hear, nothing on earth will make excess pounds melt away "like magic."

Common sense tells us all these things. Deep down inside, few of us really expect to find an easy way out, but millions of us keep right on looking, anyway. We go right on shelling out good money – to the tune of billions of dollars annually – for products we know are too good to be true. And, sure enough, they are:

"Quit smoking painlessly! Never crave a cigarette again!"

"Lose as much weight as you want with our revolutionary weight-loss plan!"

"Amazing new machine tones muscles while you sleep, without exercise!"

"Lose inches overnight from waist, thighs and buttocks!"

We've all heard the same kind of pitches over and over again. Most of us know better, but we go right on buying this stuff, anyway – anti-smoking chewing gum, spot reducing devices, diet pills and potents, magic beauty formulas, automatic exercisers, vitamins to give you super-strength.

As P. T. Barnum said, "There's a sucker born every minute." That's the only explanation I can think of for this ludicrous phenomenon.

In the final analysis, genuine self-improvement always relates back to genuine effort and motivation. If there's any compromise or substitute, I've never discovered it in all my searching. You don't have to have scads of money or wield great power and influence or possess vast scientific knowledge to enjoy good health and long life. What you do need is desire and self-discipline.

But the good news is, once you succeed in improving just one aspect of yourself, finding the will to do more becomes less difficult. Success breeds success. And there's no greater feeling of satisfaction in the world than knowing you've faced up to a long-term problem and overcome it honestly, without gimmicks, gadgets or cynically promoted "miracles."

Affordable Health Foods

In some respects, health food stores are important resources that provide a vital service. There are certain foods, supplements and other nutritional elements that can rarely, if ever, be found in mainstream supermarkets. But because health food stores now operate in virtually all cities and larger towns, these products are readily available to the vast majority of Americans.

Health food retailers have also benefitted the public by introducing a variety of previously unfamiliar products to the marketplace. Just 10 years ago, ordinary grocery chains didn't stock many of these products. Now they frequently do, and health food stores deserve a lot of the credit for this merchandising breakthrough.

But too often the health food stores have continued to charge the same high prices they charged when they were the only game in town. In most cases, there's no reason to pay those high prices anymore.

I shop in health food stores on an average of once or twice a month, but I usually don't buy any item I know I can find in the supermarket, simply because supermarket prices are almost always lower. I could understand the differences in prices if all health food stores fell into the "mom and pop" category, but they clearly don't. On the contrary, most of the health food stores in most big cities are run by national or regional chains. Some qualify as supermarkets in their own right. I see no reason why they can't offer competitive prices.

Is "Organic" Really Better?

One of the misconceptions promoted by health food retailers is the idea that only "organically grown" foods are nutritionally sound, and that foods grown with commercial fertilizers are inferior in quality. There is absolutely no reliable evidence, however, to support this contention.

Scientific analysis shows that fruits, vegetables and grains have the same nutritive value whether they are fertilized with chemicals or organic substances. I'll be the first to agree that chemical fertilizers have often been overused and the runoff from fields where they are used has added to the problem of water pollution. But that doesn't mean that a tomato grown with these fertilizers contains any less calories or nutrients than a tomato grown organically.

There's one thing that is different about these two types of food, though, and that's the price. Organic foods are always much more expensive.

In my opinion, the simplest way to get the best value when buying food is to let your senses of sight, touch, smell – and occasionally taste – be your guide. A good tomato is round and plump and bright-red, not pink or orange and flat on one side. A sweet, ripe cataloupe has a distinctive aroma about it. A good ear of corn has firm, uniform kernels that ooze milky juice when punctured by a thumbnail. And so on.

Again, it's a matter of common sense – something that no "organically grown" sign can take the place of.

When Too Much Isn't Enough

All told, more than 40 different vitamins, minerals and other nutritional elements are recognized as being essential to good health. By now, almost everyone realizes the importance of vitamins, and a large percentage of the American public takes one or more vitamin supplements daily.

Unfortunately, though, most of the tens of millions of vitamin pills, tablets and capsules that we swallow each day in this country represent only a waste of effort and money. There are two main reasons for this:

(1) Many people buy and use widely advertised "multi-vitamins" that contain only weak, low-quality synthetic substances and are too impotent to provide any real benefit. For all practical purposes, they might as well be swallowing a sugar pill.

(2) On the other extreme, a small percentage of people take huge mega-doses of certain vitamins on the assumption that more is better, but these excessive amounts have no proven value and probably aren't even absorbed by the body.

With the millions of dollars spent on vitamins and nutritional supplements, it's no wonder that the health hucksters are especially active in this area. My advice is to take reasonable quantities of vitamins and minerals. It's true that the recommended daily allowances of certain nutrients are generally too low, and it can do no harm to take 10 or 20 times as much as the RDA. But beyond that, consumers are usually throwing money away.

There's still much to be learned about how vitamins work and interact in the body. But an adequate, health-building, disease-preventing daily supply of all 40-plus key nutrients should be within most people's budget. (For my specific recommendations about daily vitamin dosages, refer back to Chapter Five.)

Do you need to buy a separate little bottle of every conceivable type of nutrient from alfalfa to zinc – the kind that normally sell for $15 to $60 each in the health food stores? I don't think so.

The health hucksters won't like it, but the odds are 10,000 to one that you'll never miss it.

*"The best physicians are Dr. Diet,
Dr. Quiet and Dr. Merryman."*
–Sydney Smith

CHAPTER 15

Rx. for 100 (or More) Healthy, Happy Years

In the preceding chapters, we've examined all the myriad aspects of the "aging disease" one at a time and discussed ways to combat each of them. Now it's time to take a look at the total package.

It's my hope and belief that this book is unique in what it offers. Many books deal in greater detail with one specific subject, such as nutrition, exercise, psychology or sexual performance. But to my knowledge, this is the only book in existence that attempts to cover the whole broad spectrum of age-associated and health-related phenomena and problems and suggest solutions. No other single volume tackles all the physical, mental, psychological, historical and socio-economic factors that spell the difference between youth and age in the way this one does.

My goal in writing this book has been to offer a blend of information, inspiration, motivational tips and experience-based recommendations that can serve as a sort of guidebook for those who seriously desire a second 50 years – or more – of active, productive, rewarding, exciting life.

Now, in this final chapter, I want to sum up, point by point and in capsule form, what I feel are the principal keys to achieving this goal.

First, though, let's take a look at a real flesh-and-blood illustration of what a total package of anti-aging strategies can accomplish when properly applied.

Celebrating 100 in Style

Ned J. celebrated his 100th birthday a few weeks ago. And notice I didn't say "observed" or "marked" or "noted" or any of those other passive terms that describe an occasion in which the honoree is incapable of actually participating. I said "celebrated," and that's exactly what I meant.

Ned didn't spend his big day vegetating in some nursing home. He wasn't lying bedridden and helpless. He wasn't an invalid who was totally dependent on others to perform even the most basic functions. Hell, no! Instead, he was laughing, joking, hugging his wife, children and grandkids and bouncing his youngest great-grandchild on his knee. He was posing for pictures, granting interviews to the local media, eating birthday cake, opening gifts and reading cards from hundreds of well-wishers around the country, including President Clinton.

In a way, Ned had been preparing for this milestone for more than 75 years. He was introduced to cigarettes and alcohol as a young doughboy in France during World War I, but at the age of 24, after returning to civilian life, he kicked both habits and never smoked or drank again. He wasn't a bodybuilder or an athlete, but he lived an active, vigorous life that included strenuous exercise almost every day. In an era in which little was known about nutrition and the damage a high-fat diet can cause, he instinctively followed a plain, spartan diet and strictly avoided rich foods. Maybe it was some kind of sixth sense that guided him, but whatever it was, it allowed him to avoid the killer diseases that struck down tens of millions of other members of his generation.

"I grew up on a farm," he says, "and I always preferred simple, natural foods to fancy ones. There was never much red meat on the table when I was a boy, so I just never cultivated much of a taste for it."

Positive Thinking – and Doing

But maybe Ned's most important anti-aging asset is his incurable optimism. He's faced more than his share of misfortune, but he's always been a positive thinker. When his first wife died, he raised three motherless children by himself. When he went broke as a country storekeeper during the Depression – mainly because he couldn't refuse to let hungry customers go without groceries, even when he knew they couldn't pay – he picked himself up and started over. He was sustained by a strong religious faith and a deep belief that most people are "basically good folks."

About six years ago, when Ned was 94, he underwent major surgery on both legs. Without the operations, the doctors said he'd soon become a total invalid. "I couldn't put up with that," he says. "I had to keep moving."

He does keep moving, too. He goes to church almost every Sunday. He enjoys dining out and socializing with relatives and friends. Last year, he logged thousands of miles of cross-country air travel. He writes and distributes a monthly newsletter for veterans. He drove his own own car until he was 98, but now allows his wife (she's 20 years younger than he is) to handle the driving chores.

Unlike so many elderly people, who have a tendency to "let themselves go" when it comes to appearance, Ned continues to enjoy looking his best. He seldom misses the chance to put on a suit and tie and mingle with people.

Like anyone who lives a long, full life, Ned has memories galore. Yet he doesn't believe in living in the past. Even at age 100, he's still looking ahead. As soon as his birthday celebration was over, he was busily planning his next big trip to a national convention of World War I veterans.

Seven Keys to Getting There

Now, I don't claim to know all the secrets of Ned's ability to live more than a century of full, productive life. There are many genetic and environmental forces that could have played a role. A bit of sheer good luck and some other intangibles are sure to figure in somewhere, too. But I can identify at least seven key lifestyle factors that Ned epitomizes – factors that undoubtedly contribute to his longevity:

– Overcoming and permanently banishing destructive habits.

– Following a nutritious, low-fat diet emphasizing simple, unrefined foods.
– Getting adequate regular amounts of physical exercise.
– Dealing decisively with medical problems affecting health and mobility.
– Maintaining a positive, upbeat psychological approach to life and its problems.
– Making an effort to keep up external appearances.
– Continuing to plan ahead and look toward the future.

It's easy to envy someone like Ned J. It's also easy to shrug and say, "Well, he's just an accident of fate," or "I'll never be so lucky!" But both reactions are pointless and self-defeating. What the rest of us really need to do is make a conscious effort to follow his example.

Many people who are roughly half Ned's age today have the opportunity and capability to duplicate his feat if they set their minds to it. If you're just now approaching 50, chances are you haven't given much thought to the idea of reaching 100. After all, it seems so far away, and there are so many things that could happen along the way. It's hard enough to figure out what's going to happen next week or next month, let alone what will take place a half-century from now.

But if you're willing to take advantage of the arsenal of anti-aging weapons at your disposal and make a serious commitment to yourself, now is exactly the time you should start thinking about it.

What are your priorities going to be as you move into your 50s? How are you going to cope with the negative, destructive elements that threaten to rob you of a big piece of your future? How capable are you of implementing positive personal changes that could give you 50 or more additional good years?

Are you going to dare to be like Ned J.? Or are you more likely to emulate another acquaintance of mine? I'll call him Ted G., and I'll leave it up to you to decide how many similarities there are between you and him.

Deterioration and Defeat

Ted just turned 51, and until the last few months, he'd never been sick a day in his life. At least, that's what he likes to say right before he launches into his sob story of misfortune, physical deterioration and spiritual defeat. Actually, of course, Ted had been neglecting and abusing his health for decades before the cumulative results finally caught up with him.

First, he began to experience severe abdominal pains, which were diagnosed as gall bladder attacks – a direct result of bad eating habits and faulty nutrition. Like countless other middle-aged Americans, Ted had developed gallstones, which are composed primarily of cholesterol. Studies show that gallstones are most frequently caused by excessive saturated fat and a shortage of Vitamins A and E in the diet. Even after stones develop, they can often be dissolved by cutting down on saturated fat and taking daily vitamin supplements.

In other words, Ted had literally "eaten himself sick" over a period of many years. But that was only the beginning.

During the extensive diagnostic tests that were run while Ted was in the hospital having his gallbladder removed, doctors also found that one of his main coronary arteries was 80 percent blocked – almost certainly because of the same high-saturated-fat diet that triggered the gall bladder attacks. His blood pressure was also high enough to cause concern.

Doctors decided that Ted's atherosclerosis wasn't bad enough to warrant bypass surgery or angioplasty, because his other coronary arteries weren't heavily obstructed – at least not yet. But since then, Ted has started having chest pains that may relate to some other problem or be entirely psychosomatic; the doctors aren't sure. Meanwhile, Ted is severely depressed, has trouble sleeping nights and is having to take anti-anxiety drugs in addition to blood pressure medication.

Ted has a good job that pays well but also involves a lot of stress. He's averaged being 25 to 40 pounds overweight ever since he was in his mid-30s. He's a confirmed couch potato, whose only regular exercise before his illness was mowing his lawn and carrying a can of beer and a bag of chips from the kitchen to the den. Now he doesn't even do the lawn anymore. On weekends, he isolates himself in front of the TV, wearing dirty sweats and a two-day growth of beard, and broods.

"I'll be on blood pressure pills the rest of my life," Ted says morosely. "The doctor told me I shouldn't eat pizza or burgers or any of the fried stuff I like, and he said I need to cut way down on salt. Right now, I'm so miserable I don't even care."

I tried to tell Ted that getting into an aerobics exercise program and losing some weight might lower his blood pressure without drugs. The accompanying reduction in his level of body fat could also prevent his atherosclerosis from getting worse, possibly even reverse it. I suggested he try to move into a less stressful work situation, plan a vacation trip with his wife and get away from the house more often to do something active outdoors. But I'm not sure he was listening to any of this; he may have been too busy feeling sorry for himself.

If I were a wagering man, I'd be more likely to bet my money on Ned J. living to 120 than I would on Ted G. making it to 65.

How about you? What are your longevity odds? Even if they look as bad as Ted's right now, there are many ways to start swinging them around in your favor.

Obviously, there can be no precise prescription for living 100 years or more. A person can follow every rule of good health and still be run down by a car or struck by lightning. And it's impossible to know what kind of disease processes we may be predisposed to because of our genetic programming. But, even so, every one of us can improve our odds. All it takes is common sense and the willingness to make a concerted, informed effort.

I predict that the 70 million men and women we classify as baby boomers will be the group that finally makes living to be 100 a commonplace event in our society. No matter how upsetting the idea may be to the social planners of the federal government, several million boomers could end up making it to the century mark. We have the scientific knowledge, technological skill and medical expertise right now to take them there. The only ingredient it takes to complete the formula is people like you. With the proper handling of the crucial areas in your life, you could be part of this historic breakthrough.

Let's go back and review those areas briefly one by one:

Nutrition – Fuel for Life

There is no truer axiom than "You are what you eat." Nutrition is the chief cornerstone on which other aspects of good health are built. Trying to improve or maintain health without proper nutrition is exactly like trying to build a house without a foundation.

If you consume vast amounts of fat, you're going to be fat. That's simply an inescapable fact. And the fat that's part of you isn't just the part you can see with the naked eye – in the form of cellulite-rippled thighs, multiple chins, flabby arms and a bulging bottom and waistline. It's also the fat molecules traveling through your bloodstream, causing cholesterol deposits to build up inside your arteries, impede the flow of blood, and eventually threaten your life.

Some fat is essential, but small amounts of fat are present in all types of food. Even plain oatmeal has three grams of fat in a typical half-cup serving. In this country, a fat shortage in the diet is virtually unthinkable.

To promote peak health and prevent the heart attacks and strokes that account for well over half of all deaths, limit your intake of fat to no more than 30 percent of the total calories you consume each day. Twenty percent is even better. As I've said before, I limit myself to 10 percent without feeling deprived.

Meanwhile, get about 50 or 60 percent of your calories from carbohydrates, with emphasis on the complex carbs found in vegetables, cereal grains, beans, potatoes, pasta, bread, etc. The other 25 to 30 percent of calories should come from protein, the best sources of which are lean meat, skinless white chicken and turkey, fish (the whiter the better) and egg whites.

These foods mean lean muscle mass instead of visible fat – and clear arteries instead of clogged ones.

Exercise – Just Do It!

Contrary to a widely held belief, people don't usually "wear out" physically as they grow older. In most cases, their bodies "rust out" from disuse. There's only one way to keep this from happening to you: Regular exercise.

To get yourself in shape for a second 50 years – and keep yourself there – you don't have to follow the kind of rigorous, time-consuming workout schedule I follow. Typically, I have four or five 60-to-90-minute workout sessions a week, but my goals are different from those of the average person. I spend a lot of that time building and toning specific muscles. My exercise program puts major emphasis on appearance as well as vitality, health and longevity.

If you're among the millions of men and women who exercise only sporadically or not at all, you'll be amazed at how little time it actually takes to increase your level of fitness dramatically. You can improve your cardiovascular health and drastically reduce your risk of having a heart attack or stroke by doing as little as 20 to 30 minutes of aerobic exercises – fast walking, jogging, stationary running, bicycling or aerobic dancing – at least three times a week.

In other words, you can take a giant step toward a second 50 years in as little as just one hour a week. (Lots of people spend more time than that just trying to decide which outfit to wear.) And what you do for exercise is less important than doing it on a regular, continuing basis.

If you want to do more, fine. Once you get attuned to an exercise schedule, you may want to add weight training in addition to aerobics. You may want to stretch your workouts from a half-hour to 45 minutes or a full hour. Eventually, you may decide to join a gym or health club. That's fine, too, but it's not essential.

Just remember: Even a little regular exercise is a whole lot better than none at all.

The Cheapest Insurance

Vitamins are the cheapest insurance you can buy against deteriorating health and premature or preventable disease.

For as little as two or three dollars a day, you can take enough vitamins and other nutritional supplements to provide a significant measure of protection against such major killers as atherosclerosis, some types of cancer and many other potentially life-shortening disease processes. Because of its powerful antioxidant qualities, I believe Vitamin E is especially important in cutting the risk of disease. And unlike some other vitamins, it's next to impossible to get enough E in the foods we eat.

Deficiencies in Vitamin D are also widespread among American adults. If you drink a lot of milk with vitamins added, you may get enough D. Otherwise a supplement is essential.

I've taken vitamins every day for 50 years, and I'm firmly convinced that they have often spelled the difference between contracting a certain illness and creating a protective shield between it and you.

If you've never taken vitamins and supplements, don't expect to feel noticeably different once you start. Don't expect a sudden high or burst of energy. That's not the way vitamins work.

In all likelihood, you won't feel any physical change at all, but your odds for good health and long life will be quietly changing in your favor.

Defusing Genetic "Bombs"

No chain is stronger than its weakest link. But somewhere in the complex chain of cells, genes and chromosomes that make up the human body, weak links may lurk that are undetectable until they begin to disintegrate and fall apart. By the time the weakness is discovered, it's too late to do anything about it.

Within our genetic makeup, each of us carries a predisposition to certain diseases and organic malfunctions. Often, our own bodies don't offer the slightest indication that anything's wrong, but sometimes a careful check of our family tree can turn up some tell-tale clues.

Do you know what caused the deaths of your grandparents and great-grandparents? If your mother and father are alive, are they suffering from some chronic or incurable illness? The answers to these questions could be crucial in preserving your own health as you move into your second 50 years. In fact, they could spell the difference in whether you survive to reach 100 or whether disease cuts you down along the way.

In my own case, as I've mentioned, my father died of Parkinson's Disease when he was only seven or eight years older than I am. Therefore, I have reason to believe that I may face increased odds of contracting Parkinson's myself. This is the primary reason why I take the wonder drug deprenyl.

At the same time, I also take several other anti-aging, anti-cancer and cognitive-enhancement drugs to give me an important edge in preventing diseases that may have more to do with genetics than with lifestyle or environment. These are diseases that have no cure once you've contracted them, so prevention is the name of the game, and I want to be on the safe side.

Depending on what sort of health problems have grown on your family tree, you may want to consider taking "wonder drugs," too.

I'm convinced that, someday, many of these drugs will be medically proven as standard prevention treatment for cancer, Parkinson's and Alzheimer's. In the meantime, if I don't fall victim to any of these disease, that will be proof enough to me that, whatever I paid for them, I got my money's worth.

Bad Habits = Slow Suicide

I had a close friend who died of liver failure at age 55. Another acquaintance suffered a fatal heart attack at 46. Still another was killed by lung cancer at 49. The wife of a former business associate dropped dead of a stroke when she was only 41.

Two of these people died suddenly, seemingly without warning. One of them lingered for months, another for several weeks, after the doctors told them it was hopeless. In every one of these cases, a different cause of death was listed on the death certificate. But in actuality, the causes were all the same. Every one of these people committed suicide – a form of suicide triggered by abusive habits and addictive behavior.

The man whose liver failed had averaged drinking a fifth of bourbon a day for three years before he died. The heart attack victim was stressed-out, sedentary, 50 pounds overweight and smoked like a blast furnace. The lung cancer patient had been a three-pack-a-day smoker for nearly 30 years. The young wife had just snorted several lines of cocaine when a blood vessel burst in her brain.

These are four cases among millions of preventable premature deaths that happen each year in this country.

Being struck down in the prime of life is always a tragedy, not only for the person who dies many years before his or her time, but for the friends and family members who are left behind to mourn and try to rationalize their loss. But the biggest tragedy is that most of these victims didn't need to die. All it took for them to stay alive was to kick a bad habit.

Face it, destructive habits kill people – lots of people. And after age 45 or 50, the dangerous effects of these habits are magnified with each passing year. A variety of deadly diseases feed on these habits. Many victims also die in car crashes, shootings, home accidents and other misadventures related to alcohol and/or drugs.

If you smoke cigarettes, stop now – today. Stop any way you can, but stop. This is the deadliest habit of all and the one that affects the most people.

If you abuse drugs and can't stop by yourself, get professional help. If you can't limit yourself to two or three drinks per day, it's time to think seriously about abstaining from alcohol altogether. Especially if you make a practice of driving after drinking.

Kicking a destructive habit is the quickest, most certain way to boost your odds of enjoying a second 50 years.

Positive vs. Negative

Optimism and positive thinking don't come easily to Americans these days. And yet, when I stop to think about it, I know there's never been a time in our history when we've had more to feel positive and optimistic about.

The human race has always had a tendency to condemn the present and long for the "good old days." But would you really want to trade today's world for that of 100 years ago? Would you rather be stuck in a traffic jam or have no cars at all? Would you be willing to spend a week crossing the country on a train instead of three hours on a jetliner? Are the problems with today's health care system really worse than not having antibiotics or reliable vaccines or modern surgical techniques?

Ninety-nine percent of the time, a positive attitude isn't something you can find in your daily newspaper or on the screen of your TV. In all probability, you can't siphon off a supply of it from your friends or neighbors or business associates whenever you feel the need.

For the most part, positive thinking is something that has to be nurtured and cultivated inside yourself. If you feel physically fit and mentally alert, it's almost impossible not to feel good about yourself. And if you feel good about yourself, it's much easier to feel good about other people and the world in general.

On the other hand, when you voice negative feelings, those feelings tend to worsen instead of getting better. You may tell yourself you're doing it to let off steam, but what you're really doing is just adding more fuel to the fire.

Try going for a whole day without expressing one negative thought. Then try going for two days, then three. When somebody asks you how you feel, say, "Great!" – even if you feel lousy. It'll probably take a lot of practice, but don't be discouraged when something negative slips out by accident. Just try to be more positive next time.

Within a few days, I think you'll begin to feel a genuine change – not so much in the rest of your world, but in yourself. Over time, you can train yourself to look for positives, rather than negatives, in whatever you encounter. When this happens, you can be more tolerant and sympathetic toward the gripers and grumpers, even though you don't join in their griping and grumping anymore.

After all, your upbeat attitude is going to allow you to live longer than they do – and you're going to have a heckuva lot more fun doing it!

More Than Skin-Deep

Take a good, hard look at yourself in the mirror, and do your best to make an objective assessment of what you see. Almost nobody has a flawless face and figure or perfect skin and hair. But how much of the image staring back at you from the glass is the product of carelessness and neglect? How much represents tell-tale signs of being out of shape and "letting yourself go"? How much is the unavoidable result of the passing years? And how much falls under the heading of "dirty tricks" by Mother Nature?

Regardless of the cause, what you need to understand is that much of what you see that you don't like is completely correctable, assuming you care enough to do something about it. Part of it you can correct yourself. The rest you can get someone else to do for you.

Proper nutrition and exercise can melt away those excess pounds and inches. Liposuction can get rid of those extra chins. A facelift can cure that sagging jawline. An implant can lift and curve that shapeless bust. Hair transplants or a hairpiece can cover that bald spot. A chemical peel can get rid of that tired, sun-damaged skin. Contact lenses can replace those saucer-sized, eye-distorting spectacles. Caps can restore those worn or broken teeth to the pearly gems they used to be.

So what are you waiting for?

Some people contend that looks are only skin-deep. But you'll never convince me of that. To me, appearance is something that affects every fiber of our being. Nothing has greater impact on the self-image we carry around with us. Personal appearance can be a tonic – or a toxin – to the spirit and the soul.

As a simple little test for yourself on how much importance you attach to appearance, take a look inside your closet. If the majority of the clothes you see have been hanging around for four or five years or more and if you don't spot a single garment that's still fresh or exciting, it's time to make some changes. It's time to pack up those tired old duds – including anything you haven't worn in a year, unless it has true sentimental value – and donate them to Goodwill. It's time to go shopping for something you'll be eager to put on the next time you go out.

When you lose the desire to appear attractive to others – particularly others of the opposite sex – you've lost something utterly irreplaceable. No one should ever outgrow the need to look his or her best. To wear nice clothes and be well-groomed. To project charm and sex appeal.

If you ever do, then you've aged in much more than looks alone.

Keeping the Fire Burning

When you were 21, your sex drive was like a roaring inferno. Its heat touched every aspect of your being and influenced the whole course of your existence. You never had to fan the flames or add fuel. On the contrary, you probably had to dampen it and hold it in check to keep it from bursting forth like a forest fire.

By the time most of us reach our 50s or 60s, however, it's a totally different story. Our sexuality can now be compared to a flickering candle. The flame is still there, but it requires attention, care, protection and occasional outside help to keep it burning properly. Otherwise, it will eventually burn itself out.

I assure you that whatever steps you have to take to keep the flame alive in your life are worth the effort. My personal goal has been to maintain, as nearly as possible, the libido of a 21-year-old. Your goal may be different. Sexual needs and desires vary greatly from individual to individual, but sexuality should always remain a part of life.

Society tends to joke about older people who still show an active interest in sex, often stereotyping them as "dirty old men" or "lecherous grannies." But men and women in their 50s, 60s, 70s, 80s and even 90s have as much right as anyone else to a satisfying, fulfilling sex life.

We no longer have to accept the myth that sexual desire must fade with age or face the dreary prospect of life without romance and physical intimacy.

Modern medical science and technology make it possible to remain sexually active as long as we live. Estrogen replacement therapy is vital for every woman past 50, and testosterone injections can keep the flame glowing brightly in over-50 males.

Sexuality and youthfulness go hand in hand. Hang onto the first and you'll never be far removed from the second.

The Art of Looking Ahead

Do you ever try to imagine where you'll be and what you'll be doing 20 years from now? When you do, is the picture that comes to mind usually a scene from your own funeral? Or have you convinced yourself it's better if you just don't think about it at all?

When you were 25 or 30 years old, your life revolved almost entirely around your hopes, dreams and plans for the future: Your next vacation. Your next automobile. Your search for Mr. Right or Ms. Right. The fine house you were going to buy someday. The promotions and raises you were going to get at work.

What about today? Are you still dreaming and hoping? Are you still planning for better times and greater accomplishments? Or does your horizon end at the vague concept of retirement and the void of uncertainty that lies beyond it?

In my own case, I'm actively planning right now for what I'm going to be doing when I'm in my 80s. For most of my adult life, I've tried to think ahead and organize my life in segments of 5, 10 or even 20 years. When I was in my 40s, I was making plans and mapping strategy for how I wanted to be living my life today, and much of that planning and strategy has turned into reality. Without it, I know I would never have accomplished as much as I have.

Now that I'm in my 60s, my approach to preparing for the future is no different. I'm setting goals and establishing priorities for the next 20 years. It's difficult – if not impossible – for me to look ahead to when I'll be 100. That's too far away at the moment. But if I fulfill my visions for what I want to do by the time I'm 80 or so, I know I'll be in a position to go on from there.

If you want to enjoy your second 50 years, looking ahead is essential. Remember, we're talking about half your life – or more. So you can't just leave everything to chance or trust to blind luck. I recommend a detailed plan for the next five to 10 years and a more general plan for the 10 years beyond that.

Do you want to continue in your career until you're 70 or 75? You might very well make branch manager or executive vice president by then. During those extra years of service, you could influence the entire direction of your company. And meanwhile, you could earn additional hundreds of thousands of dollars in income. Think of what you could do with that!

Do you want to travel? Or try your hand at a totally new career? Or pursue a lifelong interest that you've never had time for before? When you do decide to retire, don't think of it as the end of something, but the beginning of a new opportunity for challenge and reward. Stay productive. Keep looking ahead.

The years before you are an open door, not a blank wall. You're free to attempt anything you're capable of hoping, dreaming and planning for. It's up to you.

Taking Your Best Shot

Life doesn't come with a money-back guarantee, and no one can predict the distant future with total accuracy. None of us is perfect, and no plan designed by a human being is 100 percent foolproof. We all make mistakes sometimes and frequently fall short of complete success.

So I'm not claiming that if you faithfully follow every suggestion in this book, you'll automatically live for 100 years or more. But what I am saying – and what I believe with all my heart – is that, by using this book as a guide and your own happiness and well-being as a motivating force, you can give yourself the best possible chance to attain that century mark. You can take your best shot.

When you transform yourself into a total package of health-building, age-fighting and disease-preventing strategies, the odds begin to swing over in your favor from the very first day. And they grow steadily more favorable the longer you follow these strategies.

It's all within your power. All you need is common sense and commitment.

I'm committed to more than just completing my second 50 years of life. I'm also committed to enjoying each one of those years to the utmost along the way. And when I reach that goal, I'm going to celebrate my 100th birthday actively and in style. Then I'm going to decide what I want to do for the next 5 or 10 years.

My birthday party's scheduled for the fall of the year 2033, and you're invited. I hope you can drop by and join the fun and maybe have a piece of cake. It'll be fat-free and sugar-free, of course.

And, by the way, I won't need any help blowing out those 100 candles. I plan to do that all by myself.

Bibliography

Cooper, Kenneth H., M.D. *The Aerobics Way.* Philadelphia: J.B. Lippincott, 1977.

Davis, Adelle. *Let's Eat Right To Keep Fit.* New York: Harcourt, Brace, Jovanovich, 1970.

———. *Let's Get Well.* New York: Harcourt, Brace, Jovanovich, 1965.

Dean, Ward, M.D. and Morgenthaler, John. *Smart Drugs & Nutrients.* Menlo Park, CA: Health Freedom Publications, 1990.

Dean, Ward, M.D. and Morgenthaler, John, and Fowlkes, Wm. Steven. *Smart Drugs II, The Next Generation.* Menlo Park, CA: Health Freedom Publications, 1993.

Grundy, Scott, M.D. *American Heart Association Low-Fat, Low-Cholesterol Cookbook.* New York: Times Books/Random House, 1989.

Katchadourian, Herant A., M.D., and Lunde, Donald T., M.D. *Fundamentals of Human Sexuality.* New York: Holt, Rinehart and Winston, 1972.

Rathbone, Frank S., and Rathbone, Estelle. *Health and The Nature of Man.* New York: McGraw-Hill, 1971.

Schwarzenegger, Arnold. *Encyclopedia of Modern Body Building.* New York: Simon & Schuster, 1985.

The Personal Trainer Manual: The Resource for Fitness Instructors. San Diego: American Council of Exercise, 1991.

The Physician's Guide To Life Extension Drugs. Hollywood, FL: Life Extension Foundation, 1994.

Wilson, Josleen. *Guide to Cosmetic Surgery.* New York: Simon & Schuster, 1992.

Index

abdominoplasty 149
acetyl L-carnitine (ALC) 127
age-associated mental impairment (AAMI) 117
age-related mental decline (ARMD) 117
AIDS 127, 114
alcohol 51, 154, 155, 156, 158, 159, 160, 161, 162, 163, 165, 166, 167, 180, 199, 207
Alcoholics Anonymous 163
Alzheimer's Disease 79, 113, 116, 117, 118, 123, 127, 136, 190, 206
AMA 6, 79
American Association of Sex Educators, Counselors and Therapists 183
amnesia 127
amphetamines 154, 194
anemia 86
anxiety 127
arthritis 83, 84, 113, 132, 184
atherosclerosis 81, 119, 120, 128, 134, 190, 202, 203, 205
attitude 208
avocados 58
bacon 66, 70
badminton 99
baseball 99
basketball 99
beef 67, 69
benign prostate hypertrophy (BPH) 115
beta carotene 78, 80
biostim 127

blepharoplasty 149
bowling 91, 99
breast enlargement 145, 146, 149
broccoli 84
brown rice 84
calcium 78
cancer 15, 21, 55, 79, 84, 100, 115, 119, 123, 124, 125, 127, 128, 136, 138, 146, 162, 170, 190, 191, 193, 194, 205, 206, 207
carrots 84
cataracts 79, 80
cerebrovascular insufficiency 128
cheeses 59, 60, 61, 64, 70, 71, 86
chelation therapy 143, 196
chicken breasts 64, 67, 69
Chinese food 70
cholesterol 60, 61, 64, 69, 78, 82, 89, 91, 121, 138, 167, 184, 202, 204
choline (PC) 123
cigarettes 89, 131, 148, 156, 162, 164, 193, 194, 199, 207
cod-liver oil 83, 84
coffee 66, 99, 173, 175
collagen 148
constipation 21, 85
corn 63, 84, 196
cream 62, 65, 66
cycling 99, 205
dancing 90, 91, 99, 205
deprenyl 117, 118, 119, 206
depression 118, 124, 152, 193, 180
dermabrasion 147, 149
DHEA 119, 120
DHT 116

Index

diabetes 55, 79, 113, 119, 120, 127, 184, 186, 190
dopamine 118
doughnuts 59, 66
dwarfism 126, 127
eggs 60, 61, 64, 69, 71, 84, 86, 204
Eldepryl 117, 118
epilepsy 121
estrogen 135, 134, 136, 181
estrogen replacement therapy (ERT) 136, 137, 181, 216
fajitas 59, 70
fat 55, 56, 58, 59, 60, 61, 62, 63, 64, 65, 66, 67, 68, 69, 70, 71, 72, 79, 82, 84, 86, 93, 98, 100, 126, 135, 144, 145, 148, 186, 191, 193, 194, 201, 202, 203, 204, 212
fatigue 85
FDA 6, 9, 79, 81, 113, 114, 115, 120, 122, 125, 128, 136, 145, 191
fiber 84, 85
fish 56, 58, 59, 61, 66, 67, 68, 69, 71, 84, 204
folic acid 85
fruit 59, 63, 65, 71, 79, 82, 84, 196
genetics 206
golf 90, 99
gyms 37, 87, 88, 89, 94, 95, 96, 97, 98, 99, 100, 167, 205
hair-replacement surgery 147
ham 64
hamburger 67
health clubs 42, 44, 45, 85, 89, 90, 94, 95, 97, 98, 205
health food stores 57, 116, 123, 195, 196, 197
heart disease 15, 55, 61, 78, 86, 89, 113, 138, 184, 190
hematoporphyrin 122
horseshoes 99
human growth hormone (hGH) 126, 127
hydergine 121, 122
hyperforat 127
hypertension 127
impotence 116, 133, 180, 183, 184, 186
Impotence Institute of America 183
Isoprinosine 127

jelly 66
jogging 90, 94, 96, 99, 205
juice 66
junk food 54, 58, 60
KH3 122, 123, 129
Konsyl 85
leafy green vegetables 84
lecithin 123
lettuce 66
libido 135, 161, 181, 182, 186, 210
Life Extension Foundation 116, 128
lift surgery 148
liposuction 141, 144, 145, 209
lobster 68
male sexual dysfunction 180
male-pattern baldness 146
marijuana 154, 155, 158
mayonnaise 66, 70
Medicaid 6
Medicare 6
melatonin 123, 124
menopause 136, 181
mental depression 85
metabolism 91
Metamucil 85
minerals 6, 58, 78, 193, 196
multiple vitamins 85, 197
mustard 66
negativism 19, 20, 21
nervousness 86
niacinamide 85
nicotine 166
oatmeal 65, 84, 99, 204
orange juice 69
organ overgrowth 127
organic foods 196
osteoporosis 77, 84, 126, 136
oxygen free radicals 79, 121
pantothenic acid 85
Parkinson's Disease 79, 113, 116, 117, 118, 190, 206
pasta 66, 70, 71, 204
penile implants 137, 185
personal trainers 90, 97, 98
phenylethylamine 118
piracetam 120, 121
pituitary tumors 127
polyps 127
potatoes 66, 67, 71, 204

Index

Premarin 136
procaine: see KH3
Proscar 115, 116
protein 62, 63, 64, 68, 69, 71, 72, 79, 84, 85, 86, 100, 204
Pygeum 116
recreational drugs 154, 158, 168
retirement 25, 26, 29, 30, 53, 105, 108, 211, 212
rhinoplasty 149
rice 63, 66, 70, 71, 99
running 90, 93, 94, 96, 99, 205
salad 66, 70
salt 71, 133, 134
saw palmetto 115, 116
scallops 68, 70
scalp reduction 147, 149
seafood 67, 68
senile dementia 122
sex 33, 36, 132, 133, 134, 135, 136, 157, 159, 160, 178, 179, 180, 181, 182, 183, 184, 186, 187, 210
shrimp 68, 70
simvastatin 138
skim milk 64
skipping rope 91, 99
smart drugs 117
smoking 13, 33, 51, 60, 89, 111, 130, 148, 155, 156, 160, 162, 164, 166, 168, 184, 192, 193, 199, 207
soccer 99
Social Security 8, 9, 27, 28, 29, 106, 107, 108
sodium 65, 68, 69, 71, 140
spinal cord damage 86
spot reducing 98
strawberries 65
stress 15, 17, 133
stroke 55, 61, 113, 119, 128, 157, 162, 204, 207
sugar 59, 65, 66, 71, 79, 212
surgery 83, 138, 139, 145
surgery, plastic 141, 142, 143, 144, 146, 148, 149, 150, 151, 152, 153
swimming 90, 99
testosterone 134, 135, 181, 186, 187, 216
thymosin 125
toast 66

tomato 66, 196
vacuum pumps 185
vasodilators 184
Vasopressin 127
vegetables 59, 63, 67, 70, 71, 82, 84, 196, 204
vinegar 66, 69
Vitamin A 81, 82, 85
Vitamin B-1 85
Vitamin B-2 85
Vitamin B-6 85
Vitamin B-12 85, 86
Vitamin C 77, 78, 79, 80, 81, 82, 85
Vitamin D 78, 83, 84, 85, 205
Vitamin E 77, 78, 80, 82, 205
vitamins 6, 37, 58, 77, 78, 79, 80, 81, 82, 84, 85, 86, 114, 193, 195, 196, 197, 202, 205
volleyball 99
walking 18, 89, 90, 91, 92, 99, 205
water 71, 81, 167, 169, 170, 171, 172, 173, 174, 175, 176
water-skiing 99
weight training 92
wheat bran 84
wheat germ 82
white turkey 64
whole-grain bread 58, 63, 66, 71, 84
wonder drugs 14, 113, 115, 116, 117, 119, 120, 121, 122, 125, 127, 128, 206
yohimbine 186